NATURAL FAMILY PLANNING

Love & Fertility

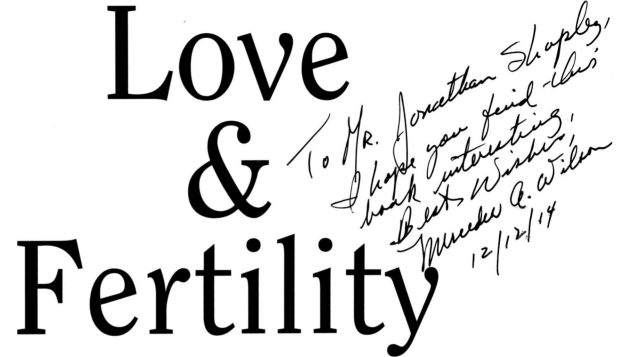

HOW TO POSTPONE OR ACHIEVE PREGNANCY...
NATURALLY!

Mercedes Arzú Wilson

Graphics and Illustrations by James Landi

© 2012 by Mercedes Arzú Wilson
Fifth Edition ISBN: 0-9633125-4-5

GW00585156

Published by Family of the Americas Foundation

Library of Congress Cataloging-in-Publication Data

Wilson, Mercedes Arzú
    Love & Fertility/by Mercedes Arzú Wilson – 5th ed.
        Includes index.
        ISBN 0-9633125-4-5

TABLE OF CONTENTS

I dedicate this new edition to my late husband and my children who have supported and promoted our work over the years. I am particularly indebted to my faithful friend and collaborator of 20 years who died tragically June 7, 2011. James Landi was responsible for much of the work and graphics in this book. We know that from heaven he continues to guide us in order to help spouses who wish to treasure their fertility as a special gift from God.

*"As soon as the word 'create' is used, God is involved, as it is impossible for human creatures to create anything. The greatness and mystery of the marital embrace, elevated to the dignity of a sacrament, reveals clearly that there is a close collaboration between God and the spouses. They can contribute to the union of the male sperm with the female egg, but they cannot create the soul. ..., the special dignity of the female body consists in the fact that God creates the soul within her body, and that, therefore, there is a direct contact between Him and her. This dignity is denied her husband. When the spouses decide to artificially prevent a conception, **they choose to exclude God** – in so doing, they no longer procreate – because the Creator is ousted. The awesome dignity of their Unio in Conspectu Dei (union in the sight of God), is purposely eliminated. They then choose to copulate like animals. For animals cannot procreate. In Natural Family Planning, God is in no way excluded: He Himself chooses to close the door to a new life."*

- Alice von Hildebrand

Foreword

One of the most significant accomplishments of the twentieth century in the field of human reproduction has been the development of a new, natural method of family planning: The Ovulation Method. This method teaches women to be aware of the unique properties of a natural secretion produced periodically throughout their reproductive years. Not only does the presence of this secretion signal fertility, it also is essential for conception.

The Ovulation Method for achieving or postponing pregnancy offers all the attributes of an 'ideal' method:

- It is simple to learn, harmless to your body, inexpensive to use and to teach.
- It is readily available and morally acceptable in conscience to everyone.
- It is highly effective in the achievement as well as in the postponement of pregnancy.
- It has been successfully used by women from a wide range of educational, social and cultural backgrounds.
- It is also successful in the various physiological conditions of the reproductive life—for example, during breast feeding and around the time of pre-menopause.
- It offers recognizable security for the postponement of pregnancy, whether the woman is currently experiencing phases of fertility or not, as when discontinuing the 'Pill'.
- It is immediately reversible and does not distort the sexual act nor involve any unhygienic or distasteful procedures.
- It does not interfere with the normal functions of the human body as do chemical and mechanical devices.
- It allows couples who achieve pregnancy to know when conception actually occurred and therefore more accurately calculate the birth date of their baby.
- It has been proven 98-99% effective in postponing pregnancy in worldwide studies as seen in the 'Scientific Support' section of this book.

This book presents powerful facts and the knowledge needed to understand the delicate and intricate functions of human fertility. Knowledge of female physiology is beneficial to everyone, especially those who are married or considering marriage.

I have seen cases where women following this method have recognized unusual cycles and have sought medical help. This often allows for detection of cervical or uterine cancer in its early stages.

A woman is only fertile approximately 100 hours per cycle during her reproductive years, whereas a man is potentially fertile every day from puberty onward. Yet most birth control devices and chemicals have been directed toward women, whose delicate organs have suffered the consequences of what some prominent scientists have called "chemical warfare against women." Men too have suffered serious consequences from some methods directed toward them, such as male sterilization. The lack of understanding of human fertility has led men and women to seek these desperate measures.

Similarly, this lack of understanding has led to barrier methods being used even during infertile times. It must be clearly understood that when artificial or barrier methods fail, it is because they were ineffective during the few fertile days of the woman's cycle—the only time pregnancy is possible.

The understanding and acceptance of the woman's short phase of fertility require only a few days of abstinence per cycle to postpone pregnancy. The couple's acceptance of the laws of nature that pertain to the wondrous gift of procreation will enhance their love and communication as they cooperate with nature for the sake of the physical and moral well being of one another. In this way, the man and the woman accept responsibility for their combined fertility.

John J. Brennan, M.D., OB-GYN
Faculty-Medical College of Wisconsin

Preface

Knowledge about our body's natural signs of fertility and infertility is just now being revealed to women even though it has been known to medicine since the 19th century.

I first learned about the natural signs of fertility in 1968 while living in Melbourne, Australia. Having read an article in the local paper about a new natural method of family planning, I visited the center where the Ovulation Method was being taught. To my amazement, in less than half an hour I learned this simple and safe method that enables a woman to postpone pregnancy without endangering her physical and emotional health with chemical agents or dangerous devices.

We were taught the scientific fact that the only time the man's sperm can survive in the woman's body is when the natural signs of fertility are present. In fact, sperm survival is dependent on the presence of a particular type of cervical mucus obvious to a woman during her fertile phase, which is about 100 hours per cycle. This simple, easily observed, natural occurrence is at the heart of the Ovulation Method of Natural Family Planning.

After learning this basic knowledge, I wondered why such vital information had not been brought to the attention of all women. I wanted to share this well kept secret with other couples.

This led me to establish the *Family of the Americas Foundation* (FAF). We began by simplifying the teaching technique so that it would be easily understood by people of different cultural levels, especially those in the developing countries where so many can't even read or write. For more than three decades, FAF has been expanding and spreading this knowledge by distributing materials and training instructors in over 100 countries, from the developing lands of Latin America, Africa and Asia (including the People's Republic of China) to the developed nations of North America and Europe.

Some day, the use of birth control chemicals and devices will become obsolete; but how many women will have paid the price? History will question the enormous corporate profits gained at the expense of women's health by birth control methods that purposely distort the normal functions of the human body.

It is important for women to know that on July 29, 2005, the World Health Organization (WHO) released a statement from its International Agency for Research on Cancer (IARC) affiliate which revealed yet another consequence of using the unnatural to interfere with nature: "The combined estrogen-progestogen oral contraceptives and combined estrogen-progestogen menopausal therapy are carcinogenic to humans (Group #1), after a thorough review of the published scientific evidence." The IARC placed the birth control method into the highest category of carcinogenicity, which is only used "when there is sufficient evidence for carcinogenicity in humans."

Tragically, combined estrogen-progestogen is the most commonly prescribed method of artificial birth control. WHO is only now conceding what had been reported several years ago by the National Cancer Institute and other scientific bodies. For several years, the chemicals in artificial methods of birth control have been increasing the risk of several types of cancer. A "significant increase" in the risk of breast cancer, as well as an increase in the risk of cervical and liver cancers was specified.

In contrast, discovering the beautifully created and delicately designed functions that govern a couple's ability to conceive enhances the intimacy of the sacrament of matrimony and deepens the love of a husband and wife. If the couple wishes to postpone pregnancy, they simply need to abstain for a few days in each cycle. For couples having difficulty conceiving, the same information can be used to recognize the optimum days of fertility when conception is most likely to occur.

There is much to be said for the wisdom of restraint. Couples have often described as joyous the renewal of intimacy that comes after a short period of abstinence. One couple called it "a new honeymoon each month" because it revitalized the mysterious attraction that drew them together in the first place. During this period of abstinence they are able to express their love and share themselves intimately in ways as diverse as the creativity of the human heart.

This book is dedicated to those who seek to live their lives in harmony with nature. It is a book of life for those who believe in life, in love that nurtures life, and in families that nurture love. For that is where our future lies.

Mercedes Arzú Wilson, President
Family of the Americas Foundation

NATURAL FAMILY PLANNING'S DRAMATIC LOW DIVORCE RATE AS COMPARED TO ARTIFICIAL BIRTH CONTROL USERS

In 2002, the first publication of Family of the Americas Foundation's unique and noteworthy study comparing the practice of Natural Family Planning (The Ovulation Method) with those who use artificial methods of birth control was published.*

The main objective of our study was to discern if couples who practice Natural Family Planning (NFP) are less likely to be divorced than those who do not. The NFP study concluded that those who responded:

- have a dramatically low (0.2%) divorce rate
- are happier and consider themselves more successful in their everyday family life
- share a more profound intimacy with their spouse
- achieve a deeper level of communication with their spouse
- attend Church more often
- preserve the family unit more responsibly

The study was compared to the two largest government sponsored surveys.** We were also able to confirm a link between the use of artificial birth control, promiscuity, higher abortion rates and divorce. Through this study we were able to demonstrate what has been asserted philosophically and morally.

Natural Family Planning fosters communication and intimate conversation between spouses as they need to be aware of their combined fertility and infertility.

In contrast, artificial birth control carries with it a substantial negative impact on the intimate dimensions of the conjugal act between the spouses. Those who have not been given this enrichment have considerably higher divorce, separation, and cohabitation rates. Marriages in violation of the Natural Law seem to be in a state of instability due to the lack of chastity within their marriage, resulting in poor communication and cooperation and the denial of mutual responsibility in the area of responsible parenthood. Those couples seem to move from marriage to separation and divorce without ever experiencing permanence in their marital vocation.

The study also showed a striking illustration of the present state of moral decadence and the prevailing confusion about right and wrong, evidenced by the replies of the two government surveys compared. On the other hand, the NFP respondents became irrefutably different (even those who had been promiscuous early in life) and most encouraging in their answers after experiencing the benefits of living in harmony with their reproductive physiology.***

It is predictable that those who respect and follow God's Law attain a closer relationship with God as they are totally dependent on His will. Drawing close to our Creator, in turn, inspires us all the more to observe His Laws as we receive graces for our physical well-being, moral strength, and spirituality.

* Wilson, Mercedes A.; "The Practice of Natural Family Planning versus the Use of Artificial Birth Control: Family, Sexual and Moral Issues." *The Catholic Social Science Review*, volume VII, November 2002, pages 185-211.
** The National Survey of Family Growth (NSFG) which was carried out by the U.S. government's National Center for Health Statistics; and the General Social Survey (GSS), conducted by the National Opinion Research Center (NORC).
*** The entire study can be read by locating the link at:
http://www.catholicsocialscientists.org/CSSR/

I.

The Ovulation Method
Natural Family Planning

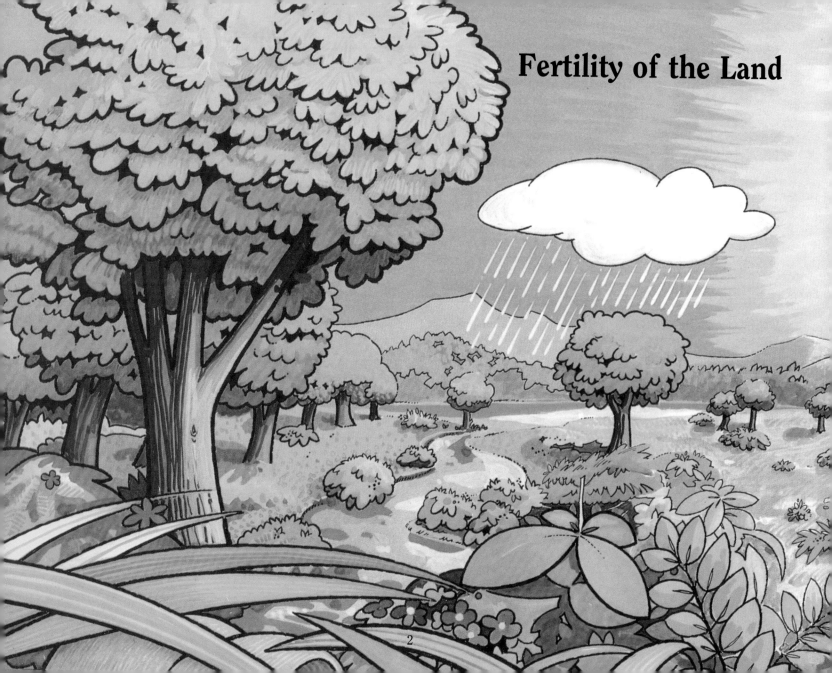

Fertility of the Land

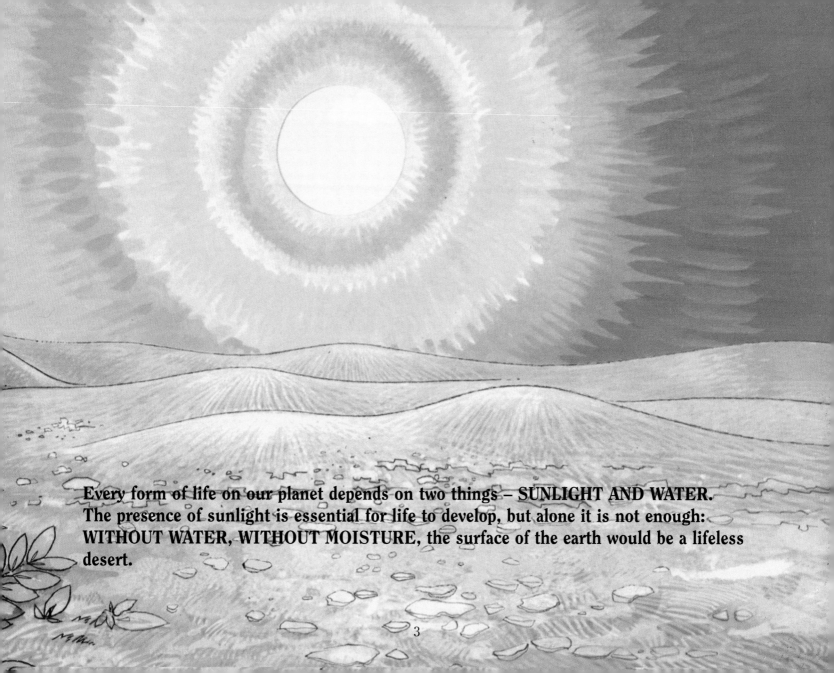

Every form of life on our planet depends on two things – SUNLIGHT AND WATER. The presence of sunlight is essential for life to develop, but alone it is not enough: WITHOUT WATER, WITHOUT MOISTURE, the surface of the earth would be a lifeless desert.

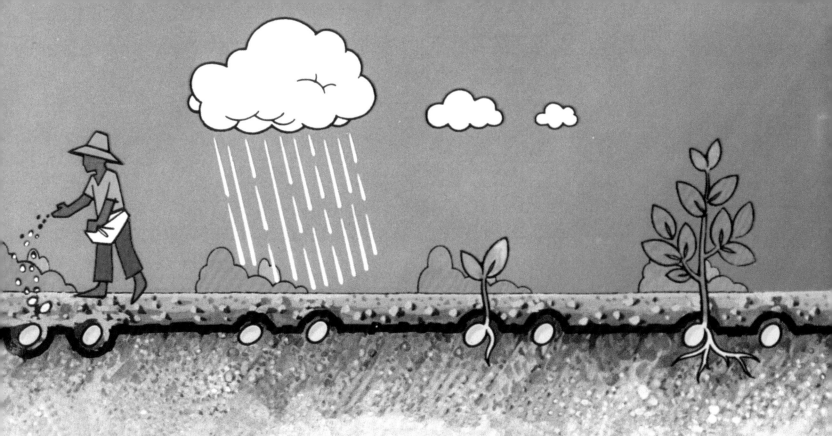

For a seed to grow we know it needs soil and generous watering. And yet, we cannot help noticing that sometimes nothing at all grows from a seed, and we wonder why...

It is not an easy question to answer; to do so, we will have to look into the mysterious factors which, like the mechanisms of a large clock, measure out the complex timing of life, the cycles of the seasons, and the rhythms of living creatures.

These same mechanisms also influence the most important rhythms which affect our bodies, especially those of the woman's reproductive cycle. Every woman carries within her a kind of clock that controls a vital function—that of giving life to a child.

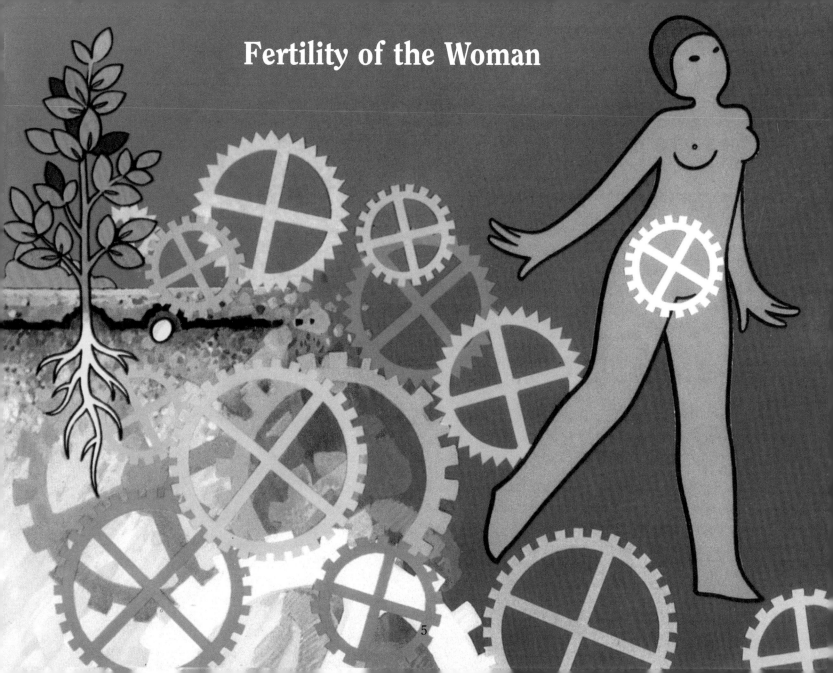

Fertility of the Woman

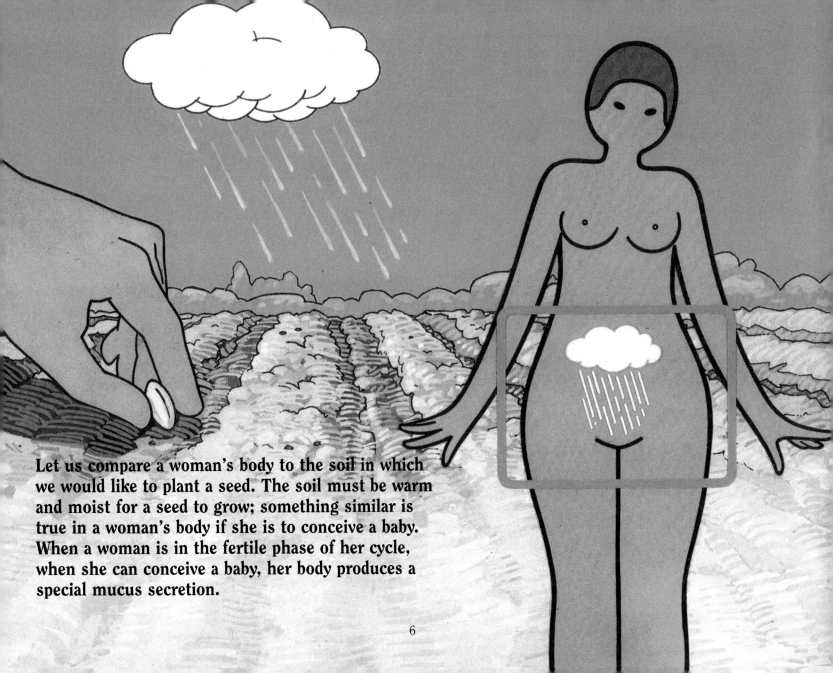

Let us compare a woman's body to the soil in which we would like to plant a seed. The soil must be warm and moist for a seed to grow; something similar is true in a woman's body if she is to conceive a baby. When a woman is in the fertile phase of her cycle, when she can conceive a baby, her body produces a special mucus secretion.

The human being, like the seed, cannot grow without moisture. As a woman goes about her daily work, she will know that her fertile phase has begun when she feels wetness and sees this mucus.

At first the mucus (Fig. 1) is cloudy and sticky...

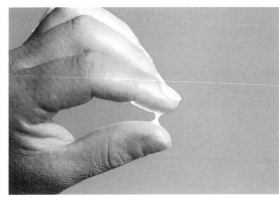

Fig. 1

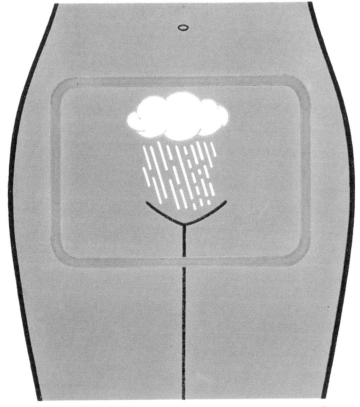

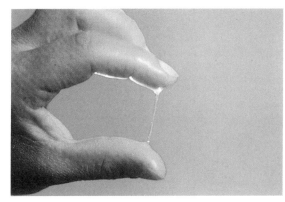

Fig. 2

then it gradually becomes clearer and more elastic (Fig. 2), and feels wet and slippery. This is the moisture we have been talking about.

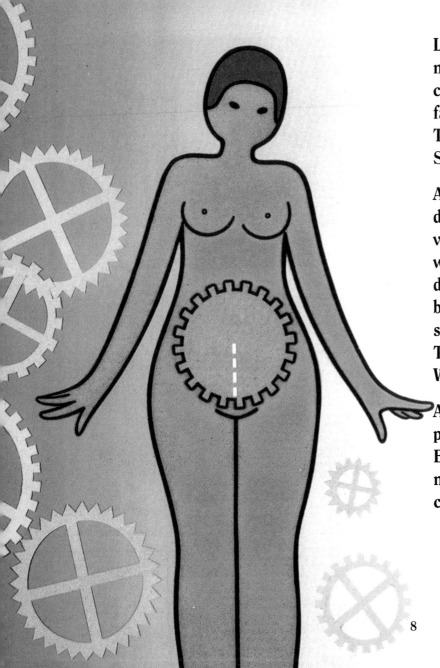

Let us now look at the phases of the woman's menstrual cycle as they are measured out by her clock. Let us take as a starting point the most familiar event to the woman, menstruation. These days of the cycle are colored with a RED STAMP (Fig. 3).

After menstruation, there is usually a time of dryness when a woman feels nothing at the vaginal opening. We mark these days of the cycle with a stamp colored BROWN (Fig. 4)... like the dry soil. Then the fertile phase of the cycle begins with the appearance of the mucus secretion which changes as the days go by. These days of the cycle are colored with a WHITE STAMP (Fig. 5).

Another time of dryness follows the fertile phase. These dry days are also colored with a BROWN STAMP (Fig. 6), and will last until the next menstruation starts which begins a new cycle.

8

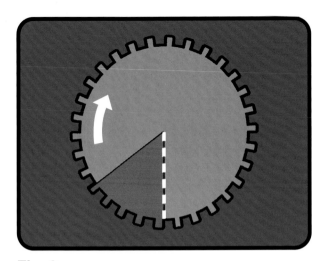

Fig. 3

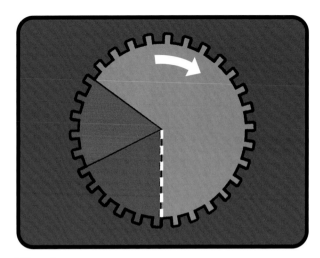

Fig. 4

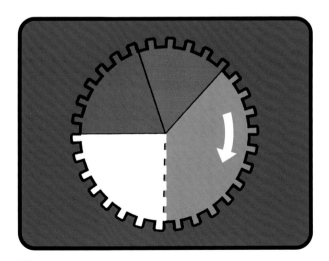

Fig. 5

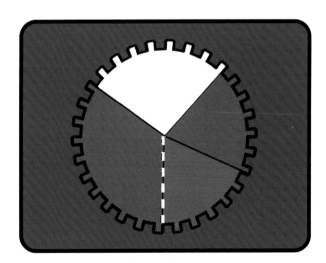

Fig. 6

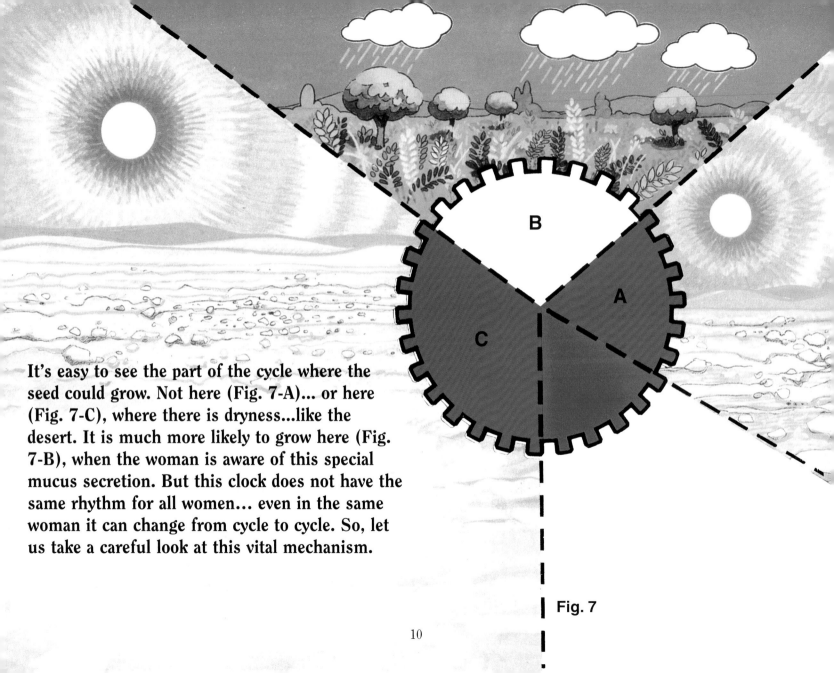

It's easy to see the part of the cycle where the seed could grow. Not here (Fig. 7-A)... or here (Fig. 7-C), where there is dryness...like the desert. It is much more likely to grow here (Fig. 7-B), when the woman is aware of this special mucus secretion. But this clock does not have the same rhythm for all women... even in the same woman it can change from cycle to cycle. So, let us take a careful look at this vital mechanism.

Fig. 7

10

We open up the mechanism of the clock, spread it out, and divide this strip into a series of 30 boxes, one for each day of a 30-day cycle. This cycle will be used again later to explain shorter or longer cycles.

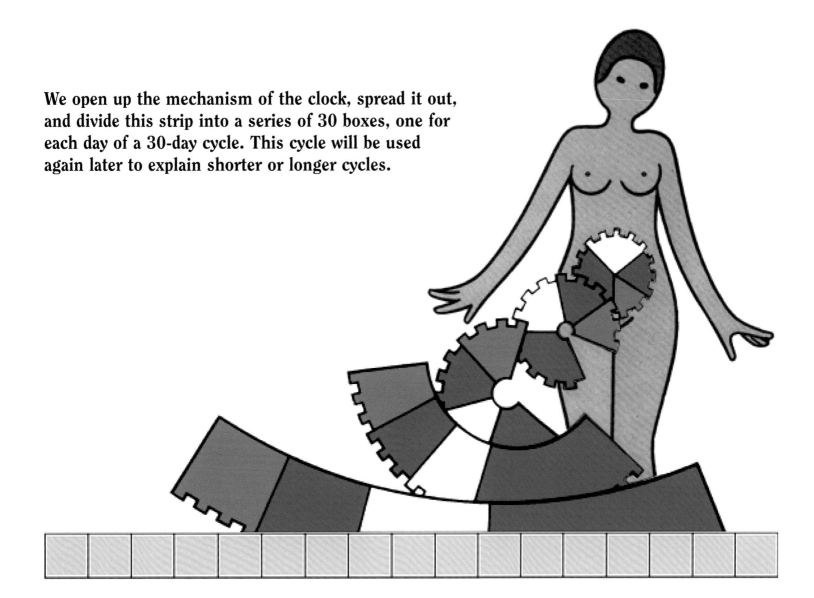

II.

Learning to Chart Your Cycle

First, we record the days of menstrual bleeding... TWO... THREE... FOUR perhaps FIVE... or SIX... These days of the cycle are colored with a RED STAMP (Fig. 8).

Fig. 8

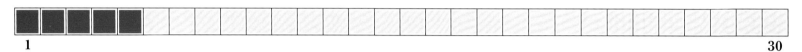

After menstruation, a dry time begins. These days of the cycle are colored with a BROWN STAMP (Fig. 9) to remind us that in the dry soil a seed cannot grow.

Fig. 9

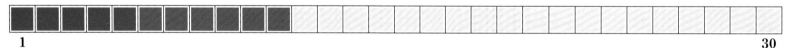

After this dry time, the fertile phase begins.
The seed can grow during these days of the mucus secretion. We color these days, in which conception is possible, with a WHITE BABY STAMP (Fig. 10).

Fig. 10

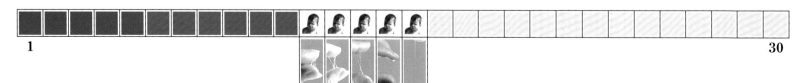

Here is a typical pattern of the mucus secretion (<u>It is not necessary to check the mucus with the fingers or to do any kind of internal examination. Its presence and changing pattern can be observed when the vaginal opening is wiped with tissue after urination</u>). The pictures on the right were taken for the sole purpose of demonstrating to the reader the elasticity and changes of the cervical secretion during the fertile phase of a woman's cycle.

At first, the mucus is sticky and dense
(Fig. 11) and may be a slightly creamy color.

As the days pass, the mucus becomes clearer, more elastic and fluid (Fig. 12-13), and feels wet and slippery, so that the woman is aware of a definite feeling of lubrication at the vaginal opening.

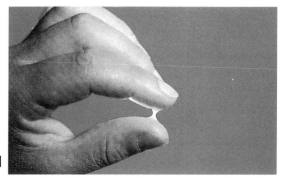

Fig. 11

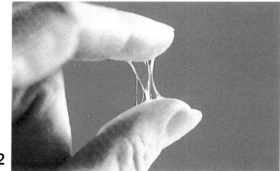

Fig. 12

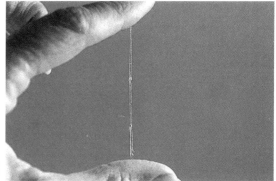

Fig. 13

Then a change takes place and the mucus becomes cloudy and sticky (Fig. 15). The wet, slippery feeling disappears altogether and the woman feels dry all day. <u>The last day on which the woman feels wet and slippery is the "PEAK DAY" (Fig. 14).</u> We mark this day in a special way (🔺) to distinguish it from all others because it is an important day by the clock which measures out a woman's cycle, the one day when she possesses her greatest degree of fertility and is most likely to conceive. <u>REMEMBER, the PEAK DAY (🔺) is identified the day after it takes place, when there has been a definite change in the mucus, and the wet, slippery sensation has disappeared altogether.</u>

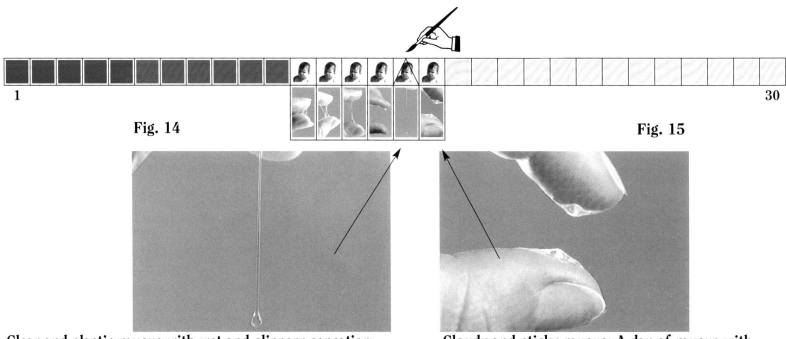

Fig. 14

Fig. 15

Clear and elastic mucus with wet and slippery sensation: Last day of mucus with fertile characteristics.	Cloudy and sticky mucus: A day of mucus with infertile characteristics

Fig. 16

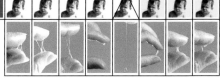

1 2 3

1   30

The three days following the PEAK DAY (Figs. 16 and 17) are also fertile days. We will explain the reason for this later. If we return to the comparison of the seed and the soil we would see that although the ground appears dry, moisture underneath might still nurture the

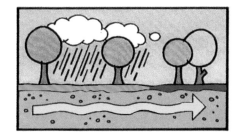

seed so that it could grow. The same is true for the woman. **There is still the possibility during these three days that sperm deposited in her body may bring about a new life.**

Fig. 17

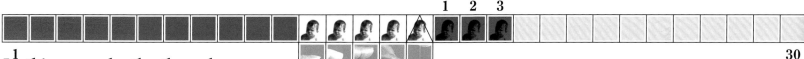

1 2 3

1   30

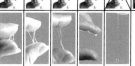

In this example, the three days following the Peak Day were dry days but they were fertile because there is still moisture inside the cervix. Just like the soil seems dry on the surface a few days after it has rained, but there is moisture underneath.

The fourth day after the PEAK DAY marks the beginning of an infertile time. During these days, without moisture, a woman cannot conceive a child (Fig. 18).

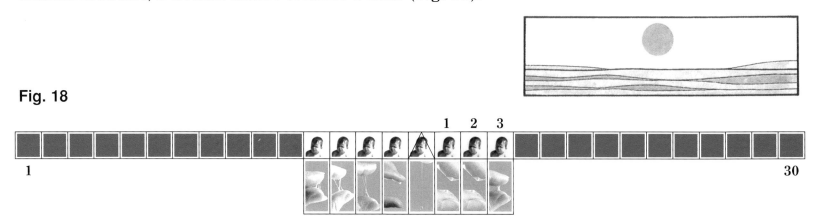

Fig. 18

Menstruation follows these infertile days, approximately 10 to 16 days after the PEAK DAY, if conception has not occurred during the fertile phase (Fig. 19).

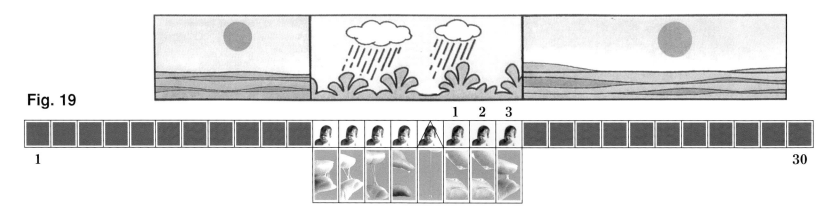

Fig. 19

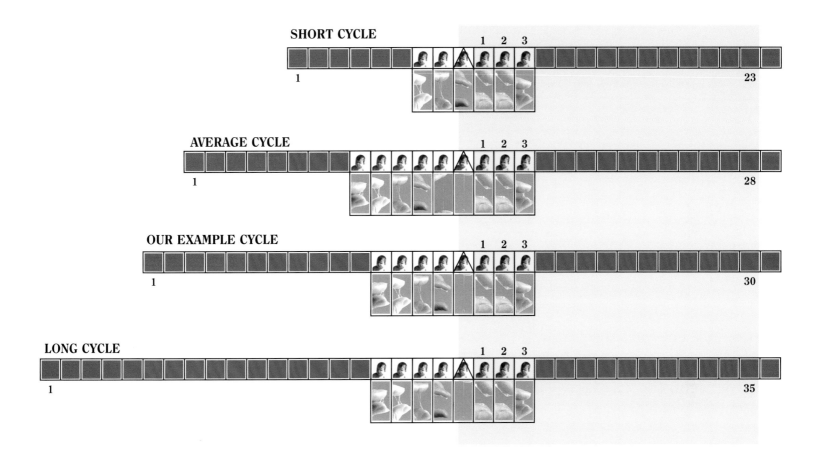

SHORT CYCLE

1   1 2 3   23

AVERAGE CYCLE

1   1 2 3   28

OUR EXAMPLE CYCLE

1   1 2 3   30

LONG CYCLE

1   1 2 3   35

THE EFFICACY OF THE METHOD DOES NOT REQUIRE REGULAR CYCLES

The time between the PEAK DAY and the beginning of menstruation is normally about two weeks. If a cycle is to be long or short, it is the number of days between the beginning of menstruation and the PEAK DAY that will vary. There may be no dry days before the mucus begins, or the dry days may go on for longer than usual...even for weeks. The number of days of menstruation and of mucus may also vary.

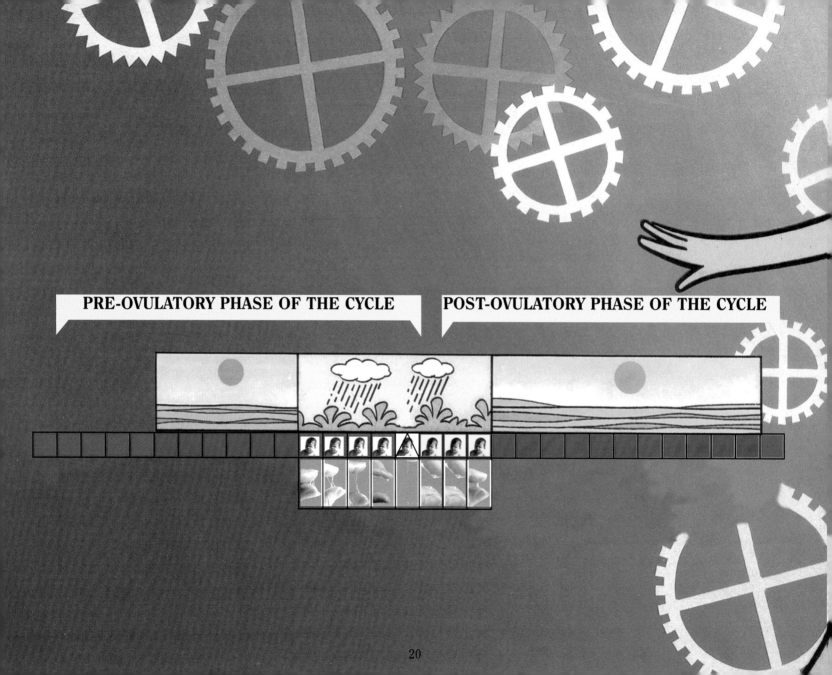

PRE-OVULATORY PHASE OF THE CYCLE

POST-OVULATORY PHASE OF THE CYCLE

20

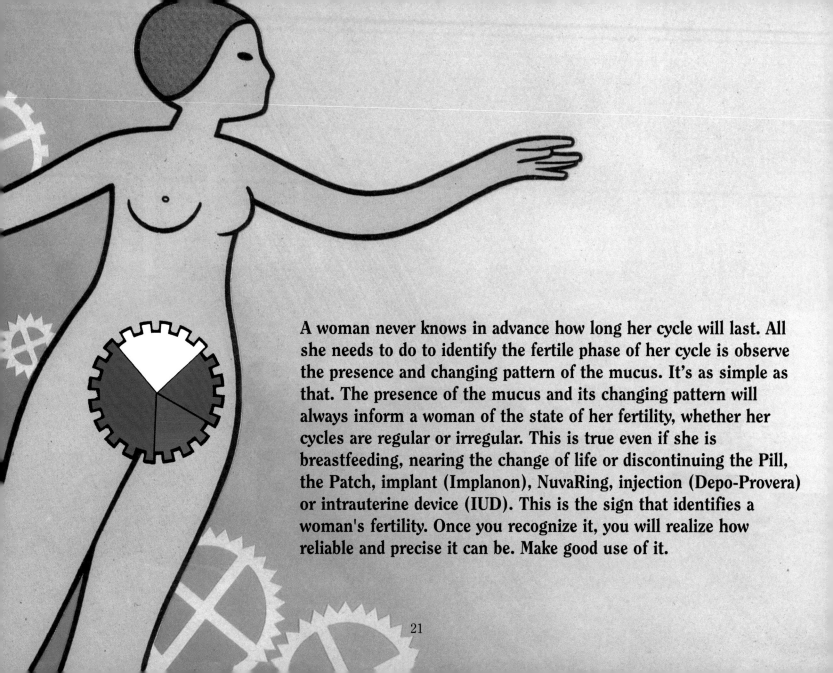

A woman never knows in advance how long her cycle will last. All she needs to do to identify the fertile phase of her cycle is observe the presence and changing pattern of the mucus. It's as simple as that. The presence of the mucus and its changing pattern will always inform a woman of the state of her fertility, whether her cycles are regular or irregular. This is true even if she is breastfeeding, nearing the change of life or discontinuing the Pill, the Patch, implant (Implanon), NuvaRing, injection (Depo-Provera) or intrauterine device (IUD). This is the sign that identifies a woman's fertility. Once you recognize it, you will realize how reliable and precise it can be. Make good use of it.

III.

The Ovulation Method and Reproductive Physiology

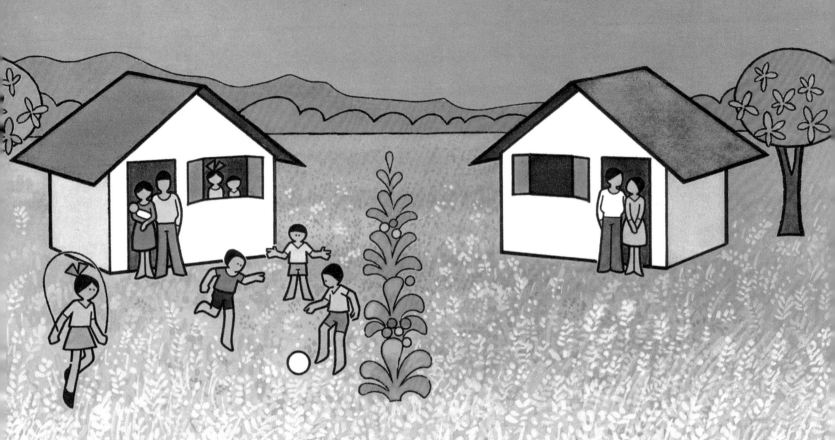

Let us imagine two houses; in each of them lives a happily married young couple. The first couple is very much in love...and their marital relationship is good. As a result, they have a number of beautiful children (by practicing the Ovulation Method, a couple can space their children responsibly in accordance with the moral and physical well-being of the family).

And what about the other couple? They too love one another but although they want children, they do not have any children. Why is that? There may be many possible answers to that question because there could be many reasons. Perhaps it is because they made love on dry days without the mucus secretion...these (Fig. 20-A), or these (Fig. 20-B).

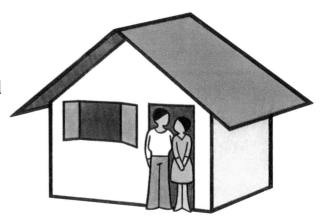

Fig. 20

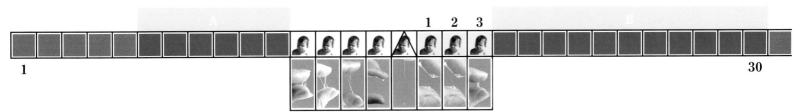

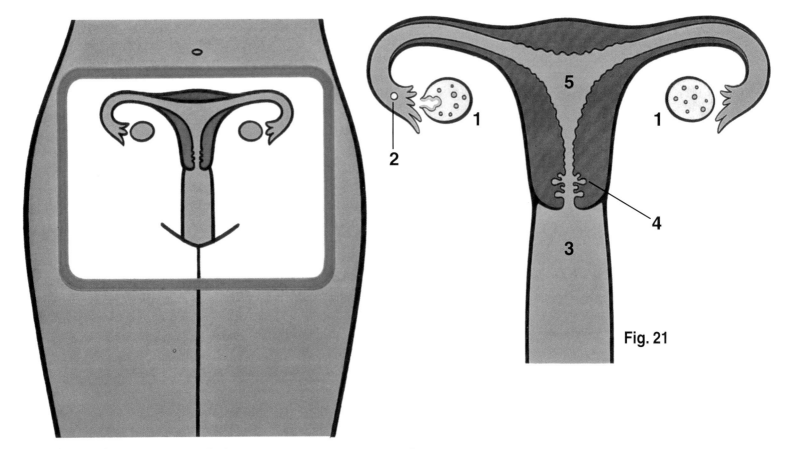

Fig. 21

But why is the presence of this mucus so important for controlling fertility? What lies behind this sign? To answer this question, let us first find out, at least in general, how a woman's reproductive system works. These are the OVARIES (Fig. 21-1), the organs that produce the ova, or egg cells (Fig. 21-2) which may unite with the sperm. Here is the VAGINA (Fig. 21-3), the CERVIX (Fig. 21-4) or neck of the womb, and the UTERUS (Fig. 21-5) or womb.

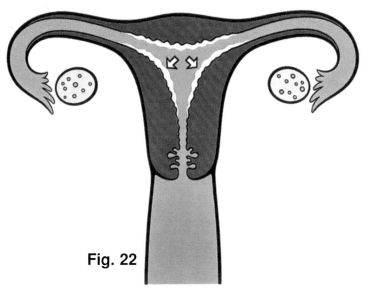

Fig. 22

The **ENDOMETRIUM** (Fig. 22) is the mucus membrane that lines the inside wall of the uterus. This lining is prepared each cycle to provide a kind of nest of tissue in which the newly conceived human life will implant in order to develop and grow. But if conception does not take place, the endometrium degenerates and is shed as menstrual bleeding at the end of the cycle (Fig. 23).

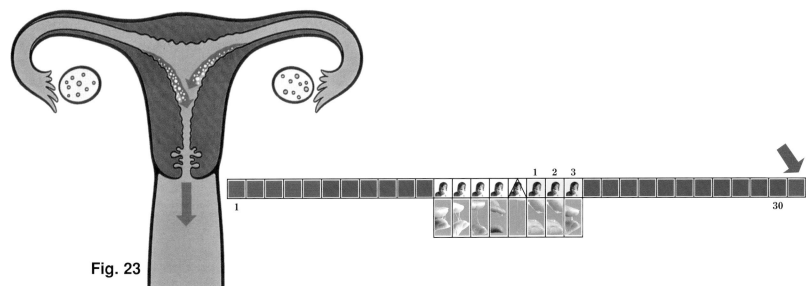

Fig. 23

The passageways for the ovum from the ovary to the uterus are the FALLOPIAN TUBES (Fig. 24-1), or simply tubes. In the ovary the ovum grows surrounded by a group of cells. This is called the FOLLICLE (Fig. 24-2).

At the start of each cycle, the brain tells the follicle to begin its maturing process, at the height of which, the ripe ovum bursts out of the follicle...this is ovulation. As the follicle matures it sends a signal to the cervix to start producing the mucus. Even the initial appearance of mucus can be accompanied by a sensation of wetness.

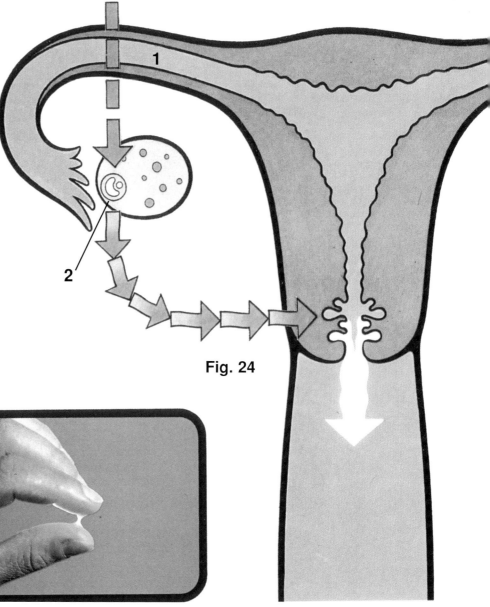

Fig. 24

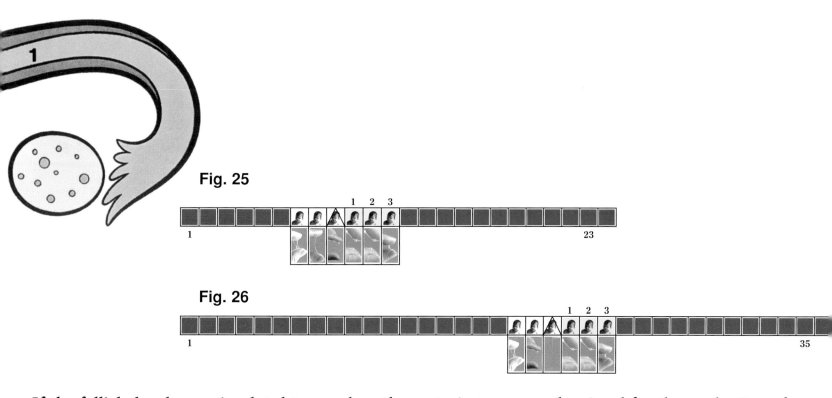

Fig. 25

Fig. 26

If the follicle has been stimulated to speed up the maturing process, the signal for the production of mucus will be sent to the cervix earlier than usual, even during menstruation. Then there will be no dry days between menstruation and the beginning of mucus. This explains why a cycle may be short (Fig. 25).

If, on the other hand, the maturing process of the follicle is delayed, the signal for the production of mucus will be sent to the cervix later than usual in the cycle. The dry days after menstruation will go on for a longer time and a long cycle will result (Fig. 26).

Let us return to our example chart of the 30-day cycle, marking the days of mucus with white stamps until the PEAK DAY.

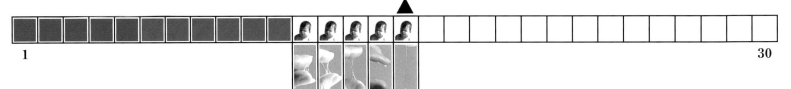

When the mucus is as fluid as this (Fig. 27) or the woman still feels wet and slippery even after the elastic mucus has disappeared, it is a signal that the follicle is about to release the ovum from the ovary (Fig. 28). In fact, the ovum is released

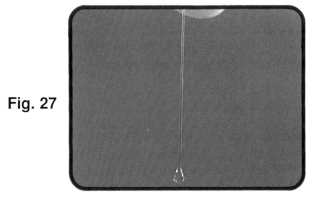

Fig. 27

around this time and enters the tube (Fig. 29).

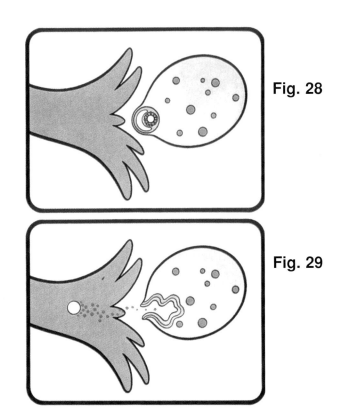

Fig. 28

Fig. 29

If there have been marital relations between the husband and wife, conception, (the union of the ovum with the sperm) would take place here (Fig. 30) in the outer part of the Fallopian tube. The time in which the ovum and sperm can meet is very short. If the ovum does not meet with the sperm during this time, it degenerates within 24 hours.

After the PEAK DAY, the mucus quickly thickens and becomes sticky, cloudy and dense. In doing this, it forms a plug (Fig. 31) at the cervix, gradually sealing it off. This happens whether or not conception has taken place. This plug helps protect the uterus and Fallopian tubes from infection. In the event of conception, the mucus plug serves as a defense against infection which could endanger the new life developing in the uterine cavity.

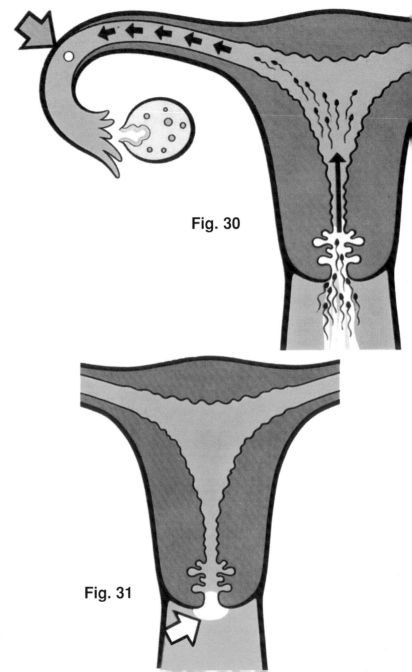

Fig. 30

Fig. 31

Therefore during the time designated by the arrows (Fig. 32), a woman cannot conceive, because the ovum has disintegrated and the mucus plug prevents the sperm from entering the uterus.

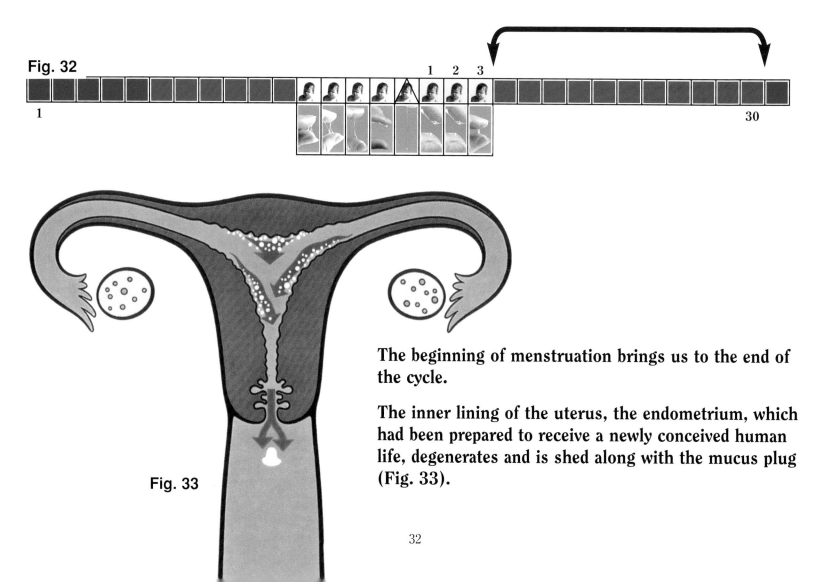

Fig. 32

1

1 2 3

30

Fig. 33

The beginning of menstruation brings us to the end of the cycle.

The inner lining of the uterus, the endometrium, which had been prepared to receive a newly conceived human life, degenerates and is shed along with the mucus plug (Fig. 33).

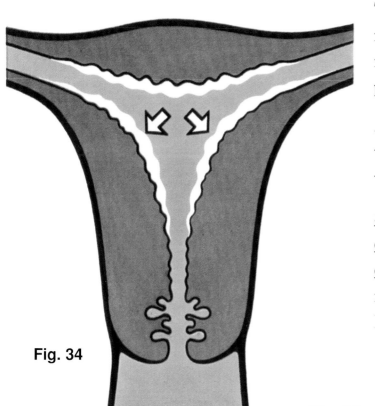

Fig. 34

This is why it is more correct to think of menstruation as the end of the cycle, but just as menstruation begins, a new cycle starts. Nature prepares a new nest inside the uterus (Fig. 34)...

...and soon the first sign of mucus will signal that the follicle with the ovum inside is maturing in the ovary (Fig. 35).

<u>Scientific studies have demonstrated that ovulation occurs normally on the PEAK DAY, or one to two days after the PEAK DAY.</u> At this moment the ovum is released and enters the Fallopian tube (Fig. 36).

Fig. 35

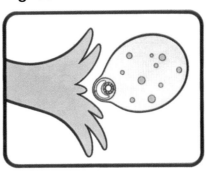

Fig. 36

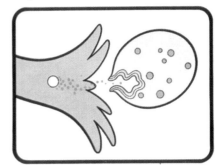

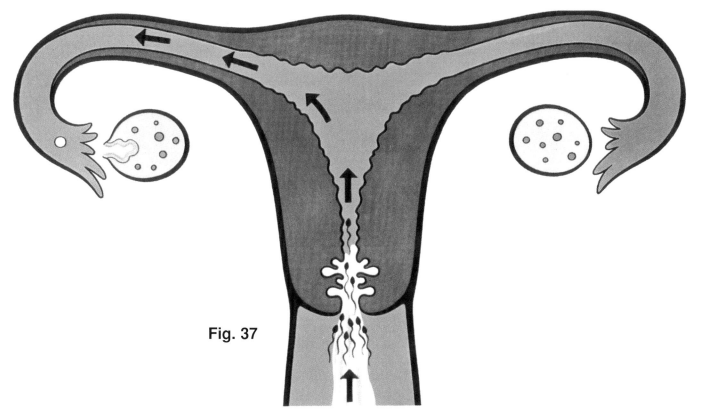

Fig. 37

Now the ovum can be reached by the sperm which have made their way up from the vagina (Fig. 37). Several hundred million sperm are normally contained in the husband's seminal fluid that is deposited in the vagina during marital relations.

The mucus filters out abnormal sperm and enables healthy ones to enter the cervix through channels or passageways...as if swimming up a river.

The mucus also nourishes the sperm so they will be full of energy and vitality when they reach the ovum in the tube.

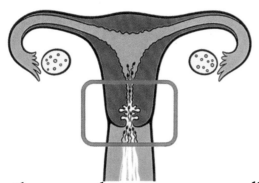

In addition, the mucus keeps some sperm alive and healthy for an average of two to three days in the cervical crypts (Fig. 38). However, some sperm have been known to live longer if the woman is producing fertile-type mucus for more than the average number of days.

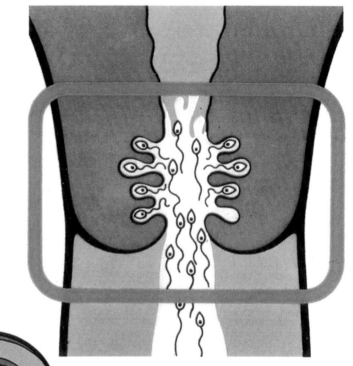

Fig. 38

Fig. 39

Now, let us follow the sperm that have gone through the uterus making their way up the tubes. They cannot know whether the ovum is to the right or left so they enter both tubes (Fig. 39).

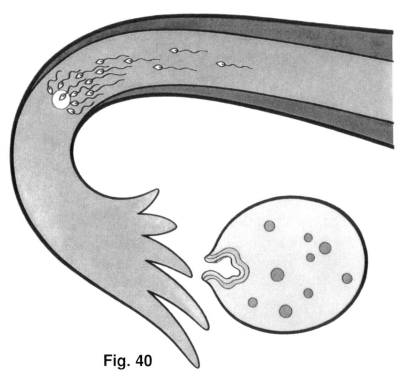

Fig. 40

Of the millions of sperm deposited in the vagina, only a few hundred will actually reach the Fallopian tubes (Fig. 40) and usually ONLY ONE will penetrate the ovum and conceive a new human life...this is the beginning of life. If twins or triplets are conceived, it will happen within the same 24 hours.

The hereditary characteristics of the parents contained in the sperm and ovum mingle and will be passed on to their child. At this moment, the individual's genetic make-up is determined. It is unique and unrepeatable, that is, it is different from that of anyone else.

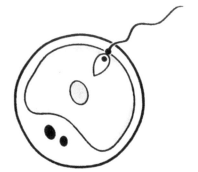
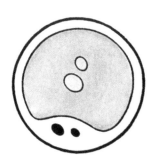
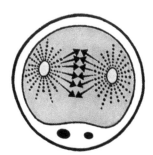

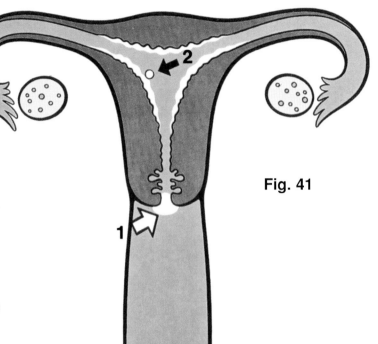

Fig. 41

Meanwhile, at the cervix, the mucus plug is being formed (Fig. 41-1).

The newly conceived human life now moves down the Fallopian tube (Fig. 41-2) to implant in the endometrial lining, the nest which has been prepared to receive it.

The new human being, originating from the fusion of the ovum and sperm, now grows through rapid multiplication of cells.

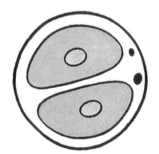 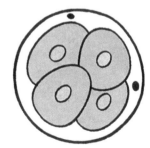 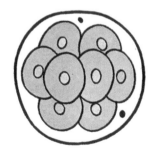 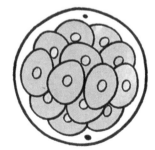

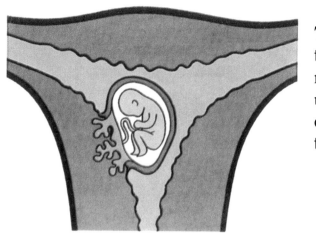

The baby begins to migrate down to the lining of the uterus where it implants, finding protection and nourishment. The developing baby will grow in the uterus for the next nine months until, at the start of labor, the mucus plug is expelled (Fig. 42) and the baby is born...

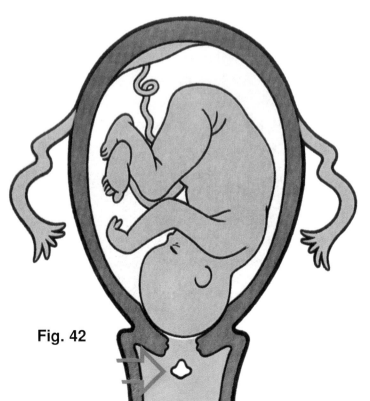

Fig. 42

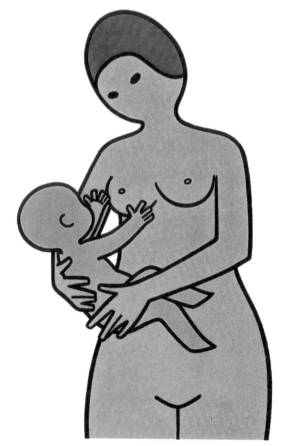

Our journey of discovery into the secrets of a woman's fertility would not be complete without a closer look at the indispensable role played by the mucus.

When it is dense and sticky, it forms a mesh so closely knit that it is a barrier even to the microscopic sperm (Fig. 43).

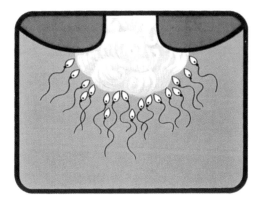

Fig. 43

As the water content increases and the mucus becomes more fluid, the mesh begins to open, allowing the sperm some passageways to go through (Fig. 44).

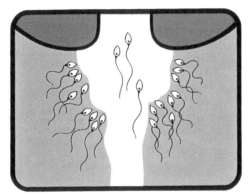

Fig. 44

As the PEAK DAY approaches, the mucus is very fluid and forms channels which "guide" the sperm into the cervix and uterine cavity (Fig. 45).

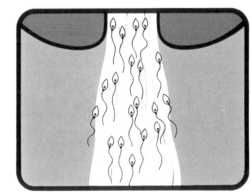

Fig. 45

Some sperm remain in the cervix (Fig. 46) waiting for the right time to travel up the Fallopian tube to meet the ovum (Fig. 47). These sperm, sheltered in cervical crypts, are kept alive and healthy because the mucus protects and nourishes them.

Some sperm will certainly reach the end of the Fallopian tube at the right moment, when the ovum is ready to be united to the sperm (conception). This explains why, when favorable mucus is present, marital relations or intimate genital contact between the husband and wife, even a few days before the release of the ovum, can result in conception.

This confirms the importance of mucus as a signal alerting a woman to her fertility.

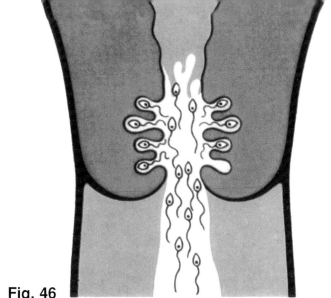

Fig. 46

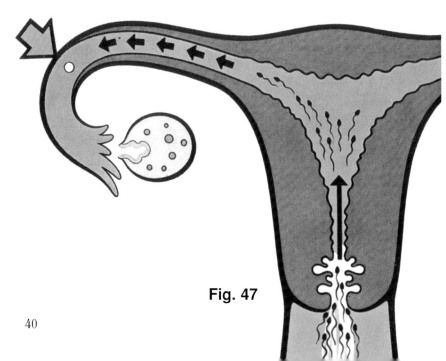

Fig. 47

40

But what about the three days after the PEAK DAY (Fig. 48)?

The PEAK DAY is the woman's signal that OVULATION (blue asterisk) is very near or has just taken place. As we mentioned before, studies have demonstrated that ovulation usually occurs on the day we mark as the PEAK DAY, or 1 to 2 days after the PEAK DAY. Once the ovum is released, it survives for only 12 to 24 hours. After the PEAK DAY, the mucus thickens and begins to form the plug, but until the plug becomes impenetrable, some of the channels formed in the mucus remain open. <u>So, if there are marital relations during the 3 days after the PEAK DAY, conception is still possible.</u>

Fig. 48

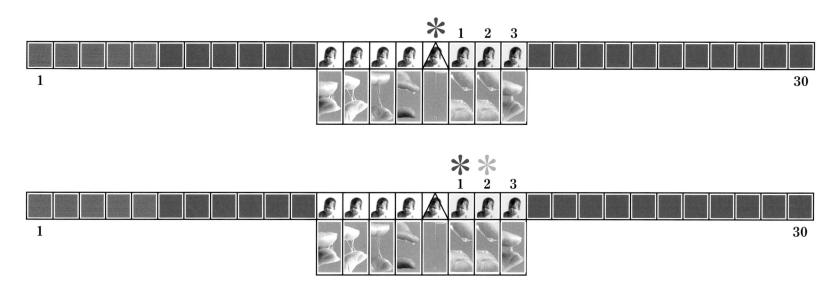

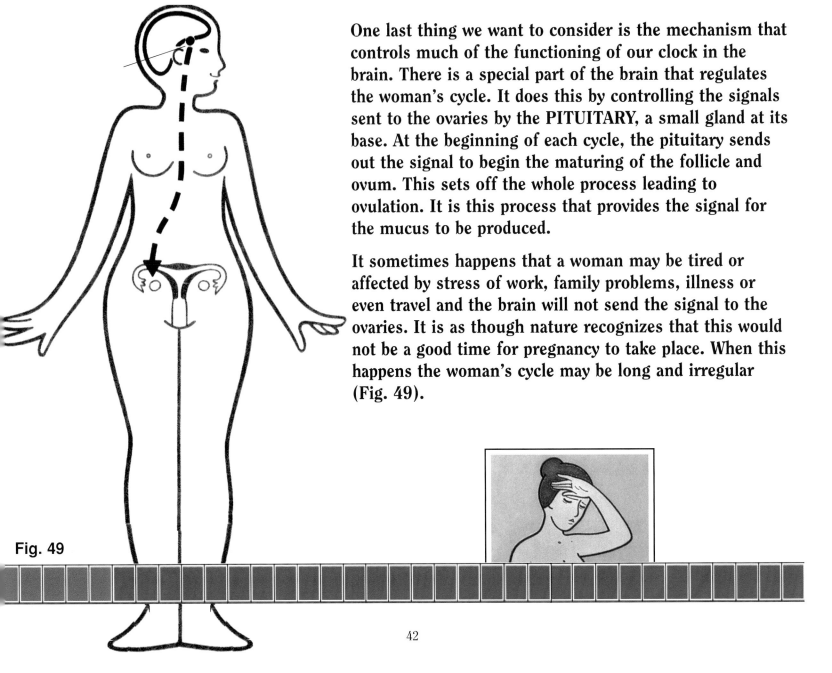

One last thing we want to consider is the mechanism that controls much of the functioning of our clock in the brain. There is a special part of the brain that regulates the woman's cycle. It does this by controlling the signals sent to the ovaries by the PITUITARY, a small gland at its base. At the beginning of each cycle, the pituitary sends out the signal to begin the maturing of the follicle and ovum. This sets off the whole process leading to ovulation. It is this process that provides the signal for the mucus to be produced.

It sometimes happens that a woman may be tired or affected by stress of work, family problems, illness or even travel and the brain will not send the signal to the ovaries. It is as though nature recognizes that this would not be a good time for pregnancy to take place. When this happens the woman's cycle may be long and irregular (Fig. 49).

Fig. 49

42

IV.

Guidelines to Achieve Pregnancy

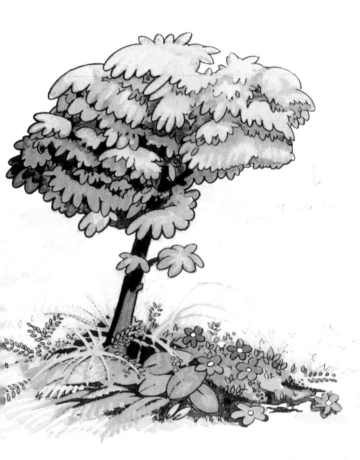

The Ovulation Method is a natural method which does not interfere with your body's natural cycles or your health.

This method is for a husband and wife who look upon their combined fertility as a gift to be cherished and protected, and the days of marital abstinence as an expression of love and maturity.

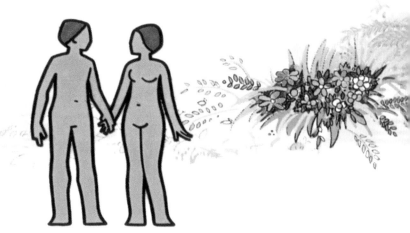

If you wish to use the Ovulation Method to achieve or postpone pregnancy, even in special circumstances such as breastfeeding or after discontinuing the Pill, implant (Implanon), injection (Depo-Provera), or intrauterine device (IUD), etc., the following pages will give you the guidelines you need to do so.

Sample Chart

This is a sample chart of a cycle. Each woman's cycle is different; therefore, you should not expect your chart to look exactly like this one. The numbers above the squares refer to the days in the cycle and not to the date. The only date that is necessary to record is the first day of menstruation. On the first day of menstruation, which begins each cycle, the couple should always start a new chart, placing a red stamp on Day 1.

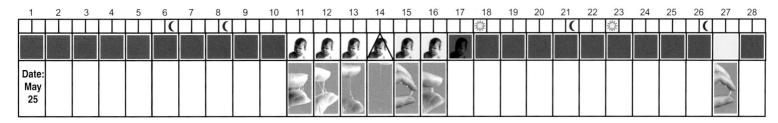

Sun and Moon — The couple themselves drew the symbols of the sun and the moon. These refer to the days when the couple had marital relations (sun=during the day, moon=at night). The couple should record each time they have marital relations before the PEAK DAY, and at least the first time they have relations after the PEAK DAY.

Red Stamps — This stamp is used on days of menstruation, bleeding or spotting. If pregnancy is to be postponed, it is recommended that marital relations are avoided during the days of menstruation. There is medical support for abstinence during menstruation.

Brown Stamps — This stamp is used during dry days. No mucus is observed, a dry sensation is felt throughout the day. A dry day is an infertile day when it occurs in the early days of the cycle before the fertile phase has begun.

White Stamps With Baby — This stamp is used on mucus days before the Peak when mucus is seen or a slippery wet sensation is felt. Chart a white baby stamp indicating that these days are fertile and pregnancy can occur if marital relations or any genital contact takes place.

Mucus Stamps — These stamps are placed below the white or yellow baby stamps when the woman observes the secretion or feels wetness. Each day she chooses the stamp that most closely resembles the secretion she observes. These are all fertile days.

White Stamp With Baby and Triangle — This stamp is used when the woman observes her PEAK DAY. The PEAK DAY is the last day that a clear, stretchy secretion is observed or a wet and slippery sensation is felt. The woman identifies her PEAK DAY the day after it occurs, because the secretion changes to either sticky and non-elastic or she no longer sees or feels any sensation of wetness or lubrication. This is a fertile day.

Yellow Stamps With Baby — These stamps are used on any of the three days of mucus after the PEAK DAY. This mucus must be sticky, thick and non-elastic, when there is no slippery or wet sensation. These three days immediately after the PEAK DAY are considered fertile. Please see pages 17, 18 and 41.

Brown Stamps With Baby — These stamps are used on any of the three days after the Peak Day if they are dry days, when no mucus is observed and a dry sensation is felt. Even though they are dry days, these three days immediately after the PEAK DAY are considered fertile. Please see page 17.

Yellow Stamp — These stamps are used when non-elastic, thick, creamy or sticky mucus appears more than three days after the Peak Day has been identified with certainty. Sometimes this stamp can also be used before the PEAK DAY, for example, in the case of a breastfeeding woman when she produces a constant, unchanging discharge day after day that she knows is different from her fertile mucus. In that case, however, at the earliest indication of any change to fertile mucus, the white stamps with the baby would be used. Please see page 66.

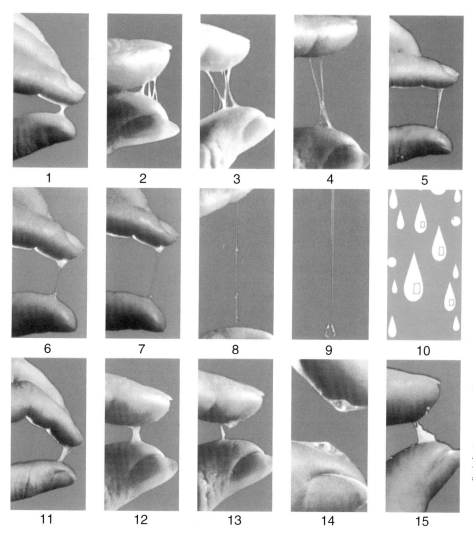

1 2 3 4 5
6 7 8 9 10
11 12 13 14 15

These are enlargements of the mucus stamps included in the record-keeping chart. The enlargements show examples of the types of mucus a woman may observe during her reproductive life. When charting, choose a stamp that most closely resembles the mucus felt or seen when wiping with tissue throughout the day. Begin charting as soon as initial instruction has been completed (in person by an experienced instructor, or after reading this book or viewing the Love & Fertility video). Begin a new row of the chart on the first day of each menstruation. Each cycle has its own pattern, so a woman's chart will show slight variations from cycle to cycle. Three to four phone calls/visits to an experienced instructor for individual follow-up and chart review are recommended when learning the Ovulation Method.

<u>Every evening, chart the most fertile sign you have seen or felt throughout the day.</u>

NOTES:

1. Abstinence from marital relations and from all genital contact is recommended for 2 to 4 weeks while the couple is learning the Ovulation Method, so the woman may clearly observe her pattern of fertility.

2. The stamps should be placed on the chart every night before going to sleep.

3. The woman should be aware throughout the day of the sensation of wetness or dryness at the vaginal opening, and of the presence of any visible mucus secretion. At the end of the day the couple should chart the most fertile sign that was either felt or seen, throughout the day.

4. **IMPORTANT!** The couple would have used this stamp if there had been any days when the woman had felt a sensation of wetness but had not observed any secretion. Such a day is considered a fertile day because the mucus is present but may be so watery she is unable to observe it. <u>This is why what the woman feels is just as important as what she sees.</u>

5. Some other observations that are helpful for a woman to record on her chart are: abdominal pain that occurs at the time of ovulation, breast tenderness, days of unusual stress, and days of sickness when medication was taken.

6. On fertile days, pregnancy can result not only from marital relations, but from any genital contact.

7. Women who are breastfeeding, premenopausal, discontinuing the Pill, implant, Depo-Provera, the Patch, or the IUD, or who have difficulty conceiving, follow special applications of the rules included in this book or the instructor will provide them.

Cervical Mucus

Cervical mucus is vital if conception is going to take place. This remarkable substance nourishes and protects the sperm and also provides a pathway for them into the uterus where they find their way into the Fallopian tubes where conception occurs. Basically there are 3 types of cervical mucus: G, L and S. Each sample of mucus is always a combination of the three different types, but one predominates. The following pictures are only examples of the different types of predominant mucus. **Finger touching is unnecessary and should be avoided, except for teaching purposes as used throughout the book.**

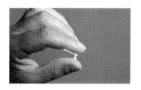 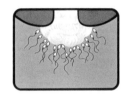 **Type G** mucus is thick and sticky. It predominates after menstruation if there are dry days, making a plug in the cervix and it does not come down until the fertile phase begins.

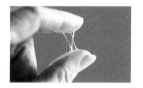 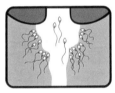 **Type L (Loaf)** mucus is a soft translucent gel, that becomes a little bit more elastic. It helps sperm climb up to the uterus and it also acts as a filter in which immature, aged or otherwise abnormal sperm cells are prevented from entering the uterine cavity.

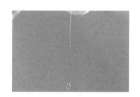 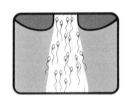 **Type S (String)** mucus is a clear, stretchy, slippery and watery secretion which occurs a couple of days before and up to the day of ovulation. It nourishes the sperm cells and provides the pathway through the cervical canal into the uterine cavity.

The combined types L and S mucus compose the most fertile mucus secretion. The peak symptom of mucus coincides with the last day of the slippery sensation. **It is important to recognize that it is not the quantity but the quality and sensation that determine the Peak of fertility.**

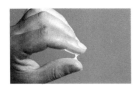 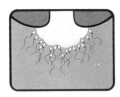 **Type G** mucus returns and forms a plug in the cervix after ovulation occurs, making an impenetrable barrier to the sperm so that by the end of the full third day after Peak Day, sperm are prevented from entering the uterine cavity. Please see page 31.

Age, Pregnancy and the Pill, the Patch, Implant, *Depo-provera*, *Nuva-ring*, Intrauterine Devices, etc.

The cervix of the woman is composed of tiny crypts that produce different kinds of mucus secretions. They are called: S, L and G crypts. In young women around puberty, S crypts are very numerous. Normally they are replaced by L crypts, and at pre-menopause, the number of S crypts is considerably reduced. Aging of the cervix is partially reversed by changes during pregnancy, but is partially accelerated by the Pill. These circumstances may be simply stated by the expression: **A pregnancy rejuvenates the cervix by 2 to 3 years, but for each year the pill is taken, the cervix ages by an extra year.** If a woman takes the Pill for 10 to 15 years and then stops taking it in order to achieve pregnancy, she may encounter some difficulties. Studies indicate that the number of S crypts are very few and, also the cervical canal will be very narrow.*

---

* "The Discovery of Different Types of Cervical Mucus and the Billings Ovulation Method", Professor Erik Odeblad, *Bulletin of the Natural Family Council of Victoria*, ISSN 0321-7567, Vol 21 No 3 September 1994, p. 3-35.

Representative profile of cervical crypts of a woman who goes through life with four pregnancies and no use of the pill.

Representative profile of cervical crypts of a woman who goes through life without pregnancy and used the pill for ten years.

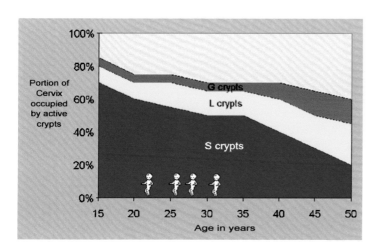

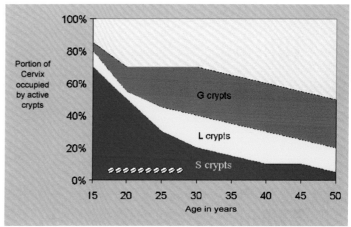

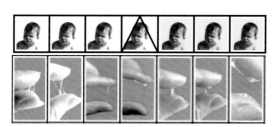

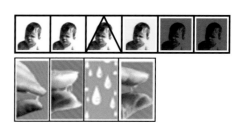

51

TO ACHIEVE PREGNANCY

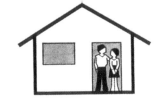

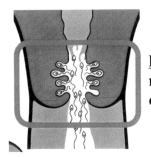

IF THE COUPLE WISHES TO CONCEIVE, they now know that pregnancy is possible once the mucus has begun and the most favorable time for conception is when the secretion has become clear, stretchy and elastic and she feels the sensation of wetness and lubrication.

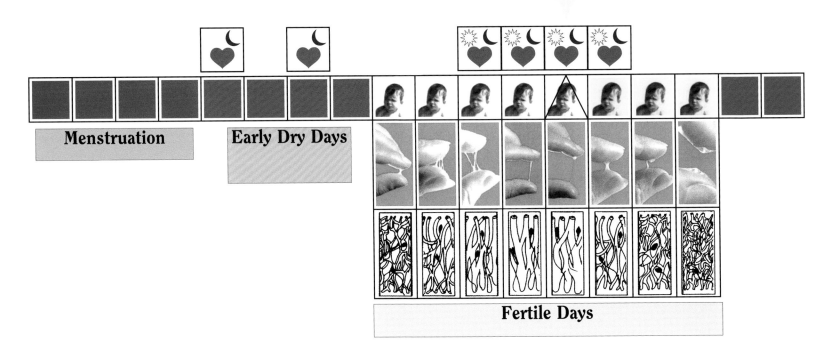

Peak Day

Menstruation

Early Dry Days

Fertile Days

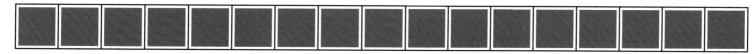

Late Dry Days

The Ovulation Method can be used to help couples by assisting them to identify their days of maximum fertility in each cycle. Most couples are unaware of the significance of the cervical mucus secretion in achieving pregnancy. Once a woman has learned to identify her fertile days, a couple of normal fertility can usually achieve pregnancy within three cycles.

Conception is possible on any day after the mucus begins, but is most probable when the clear, elastic mucus is present and feels wet and slippery.

1. Watch for the beginning of mucus as menstrual bleeding diminishes, in case there are no dry days after menstruation (this situation would occur when a woman has short cycles).

2. Restrict marital relations to every two or three days after menstruation. This is to ensure a good quality and quantity of sperm when the mucus develops its most fertile characteristics. Once the fertile phase begins, delay marital relations until the mucus becomes elastic, wet and slippery.

3. Some women do not see the clear and elastic characteristics of the mucus, but experience fertility only as a wet, slippery sensation. This is a fertile sign and the couple should use those days to achieve pregnancy.

4. A few women experience the fertile characteristics of the mucus for only a few hours. This observation is often made in the morning. In this circumstance the couple should time marital relations to take place that morning or when the fertile characteristics of the mucus are present at any other time of the day. It is important to remember that men produce fresh sperm every two or three days and therefore should plan accordingly by spacing marital relations every two or three days during the fertile phase.

5. If menstruation does not begin by the 16th day after the Peak Day has been identified, pregnancy has probably been achieved. If menstrual bleeding begins in less than 10 days after the Peak Day is identified, it may indicate that it was an infertile cycle.

FACTORS WHICH AFFECT FERTILITY:

- **WEIGHT** - Proper weight for size and body type should be maintained. Extremes of weight may be a factor in infertility. Being underweight even by ten pounds can affect the woman's cycle.

- **NUTRITION** - Good nutrition for both the husband and wife is a requirement for maximum fertility. This includes adequate calorie intake, a well-balanced diet including supplementary vitamins and minerals. Excess caffeine, alcohol, and all amphetamines are to be avoided.

- **EXERCISE** - Adequate exercise provides a sense of well being and promotes health. **Excessive exercise, however, may affect fertility by inhibiting ovulation and/or diminishing the amount of fertile mucus being produced by the woman.** Decreasing the amount of running or jogging, for example, may be helpful when attempting to achieve pregnancy.

- **STRESS** - Stress is a significant inhibitor of ovulation and mucus production in women and it may decrease both the quality and quantity of sperm in men. Coping with the possibility of infertility can cause an enormous amount of stress for the couple, but sharing the causes and effects of stress on their lives is often helpful in alleviating the stress they feel.

- **HEAT** - It is known that heat affects sperm production. Infertility in the man may be affected by extremely hot baths or showers, by close fitting underwear which draws the testicles close to the body, as well as certain occupations requiring prolonged work under high temperatures.

- **DRUGS AND MEDICATIONS** - Many types of medications and drugs can affect fertility. Certain medications such as those used to adjust moods, some tranquilizers, antidepressants, and mood elevators, depress sperm production or render a man temporarily impotent. The prolonged use of marijuana decreases sexual performance and impairs the quality of sperm. Alcohol has a similar effect.

- **MEDICAL CONDITIONS** - Infertility in the woman might be caused by a number of conditions that can best be assessed and treated medically, such as a past history of pelvic infection, endometriosis, elevated prolactin levels, or other hormonal imbalances.

- **CERVICAL TREATMENTS -** Radical treatment of the cervix with electric cautery and sometimes cryosurgery is a significant factor in the woman's past medical history. It may account for a decrease in mucus, therefore, a reduction of her fertility.

SIDE EFFECTS FROM THE USE OF ARTIFICIAL BIRTH CONTROL

- **The Birth Control Pill -** The Pill has a long history of affecting fertility when its use is discontinued. Infertility for 3-6 months after taking the last pill should not be considered unusual, especially if the woman's cycles were irregular prior to taking the Pill. However, if the woman has been on the pill for several years, her fertility may not return in a year or more. Levels of vitamins B2, B6, B12, Vitamin C and folic acid are lower in Pill users than in women who do not take the Pill; Vitamin A levels are elevated, as are iron and copper levels. It is possible that vitamin supplements of minimum daily requirements of vitamins B2, B6, B12, C, E, and folic acid may assist the woman's return to fertility.

Women discontinuing the Pill often experience a continuous mucus discharge, which will usually slowly disappear, although it may persist for 2 to 3 years. If a woman has a continuous discharge after discontinuing the Pill, she should observe carefully for any change in the discharge such as in its elasticity or in the sensation it produces which would indicate possible fertility. An unchanging discharge indicates infertility. It is also recommended that a couple wait at least 3-6 months after discontinuing the Pill before attempting to achieve pregnancy. This is to allow the woman's body time to return to normal and give her natural cycle a chance to reestablish itself.

- **Intrauterine Device (I.U.D.)** - The IUD is a foreign object inserted in the uterus which creates an environment for inflammation within the uterine cavity. This chronic inflammation of the endometrium, or lining of the uterus, prevents implantation of a newly conceived human life, therefore; it acts as an abortifacient. The IUD's string, which extends through the cervix, can act as a wick for bacteria and can cause a constant irritation to the cervix which influences its capacity to produce good quality mucus. Many IUD users develop some form of pelvic infection that may potentially affect their fertility.

Please, read pages 140-148 for more detailed information about the effects on fertility after using artificial methods of birth control.

The Ovulation Method can be used to help couples achieve pregnancy by assisting them to identify their days of maximum fertility in each cycle. Below is an example of a woman's cycle in which the couple wanted to achieve pregnancy. Whether the couple has had problems conceiving or not, it is recommended that they have marital relations every two to three days, prior to the fertile phase, because men produce fresh sperm every two to three days.

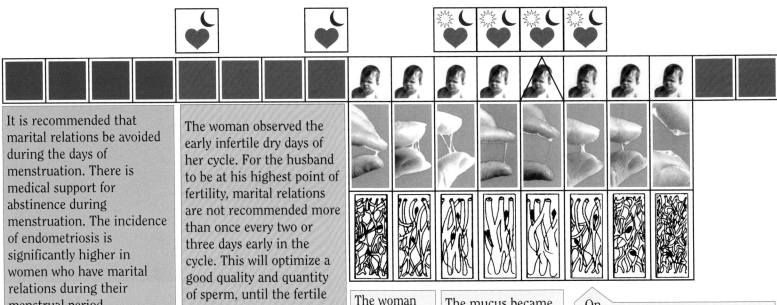

It is recommended that marital relations be avoided during the days of menstruation. There is medical support for abstinence during menstruation. The incidence of endometriosis is significantly higher in women who have marital relations during their menstrual period. Endometriosis increases probability of infertility as a result of the inflammatory process associated with it.*

* Filer, Robert and Wu Chung, "Coitus During Menses: Its effect on endometriosis & Pelvic Inflammatory disease," *Journal of Reproductive Medicine*, November, 1989; p. 887-890.

The woman observed the early infertile dry days of her cycle. For the husband to be at his highest point of fertility, marital relations are not recommended more than once every two or three days early in the cycle. This will optimize a good quality and quantity of sperm, until the fertile phase begins.

The woman observed sticky, cloudy mucus which became clearer and more elastic. The couple delayed marital relations until the days with the most fertile characteristics of the mucus appeared.

The mucus became more elastic, she felt wetness and a lubricative sensation. The couple used these days and the day after to achieve pregnancy.

On this day, she noticed the change from fertile type mucus to sticky, non-stretchy. The sensation of wetness and lubrication also disappeared. Therefore the day before was the Peak of her fertility.

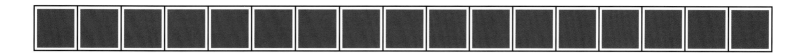

Guidelines for Achieving Pregnancy

Conception is possible on any day after the mucus begins.
Conception is *most* probable on days of clear, stretchy mucus which is accompanied by a wet, lubricative sensation.

Special Considerations:

—A couple who uses the Ovulation Method to achieve pregnancy and who has no history of infertility could be advised to have marital relations whenever they wish, once the mucus begins.
—A couple who wishes to maximize their chance of pregnancy in their first cycle should make sure they have marital relations on the days when the most fertile characteristics of the mucus are present.

- When there are short durations of mucus with fertile characteristics (Types L and S as seen on page 49)

Some women find it difficult to conceive because they have very few days of mucus with fertile characteristics that sometimes lasts only a few hours in one day. This is an example of a woman's cycle in which mucus with fertile characteristics was observed only as a sensation of wetness for two days.

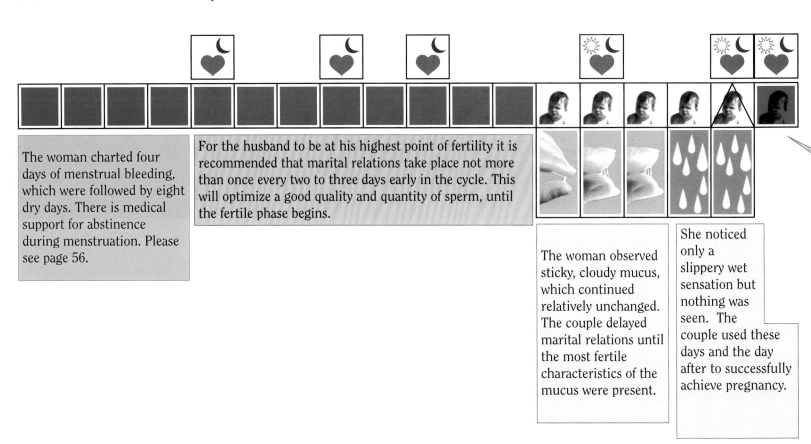

The woman charted four days of menstrual bleeding, which were followed by eight dry days. There is medical support for abstinence during menstruation. Please see page 56.

For the husband to be at his highest point of fertility it is recommended that marital relations take place not more than once every two to three days early in the cycle. This will optimize a good quality and quantity of sperm, until the fertile phase begins.

The woman observed sticky, cloudy mucus, which continued relatively unchanged. The couple delayed marital relations until the most fertile characteristics of the mucus were present.

She noticed only a slippery wet sensation but nothing was seen. The couple used these days and the day after to successfully achieve pregnancy.

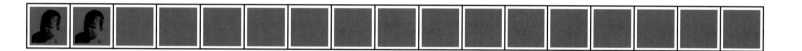

On the eighteenth day she observed a return to dryness which signaled that the PEAK DAY was on the previous day.

-When small amounts of mucus are produced

Some women find it difficult to conceive because small amounts of mucus are produced by the cervical crypts. This is an example of a woman's cycle in which small amounts of mucus were produced.

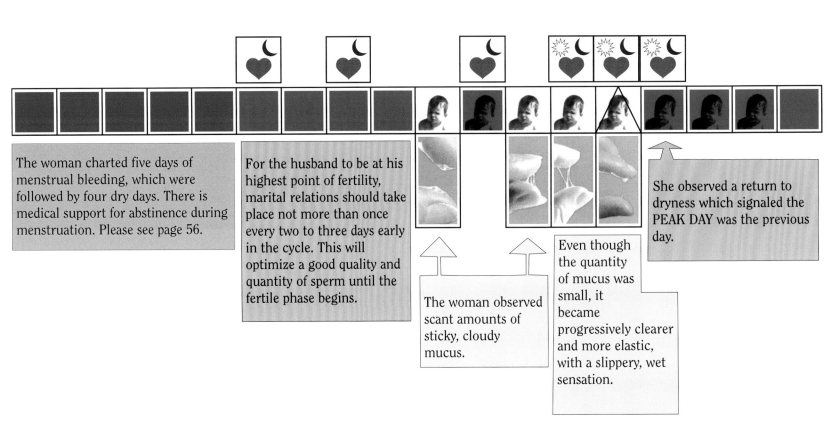

The woman charted five days of menstrual bleeding, which were followed by four dry days. There is medical support for abstinence during menstruation. Please see page 56.

For the husband to be at his highest point of fertility, marital relations should take place not more than once every two to three days early in the cycle. This will optimize a good quality and quantity of sperm until the fertile phase begins.

The woman observed scant amounts of sticky, cloudy mucus.

Even though the quantity of mucus was small, it became progressively clearer and more elastic, with a slippery, wet sensation.

She observed a return to dryness which signaled the PEAK DAY was the previous day.

The remaining days of her cycle were characterized by dryness.

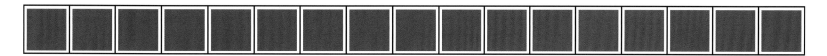

> **Important:**
> The woman was aware that she produced very small amounts of mucus, so <u>she observed carefully for the quality and sensation of mucus, not the quantity</u>. The couple delayed marital relations until the most fertile characteristics of the mucus were present and used those two days and the day after to achieve pregnancy.

THE GENDER OF A GIRL OR A BOY

Men and Women have 46 Chromosomes;
2 of them are sex chromosomes.

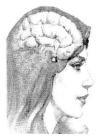

FEMALE
In the woman
the two sex chromosomes
are XX.

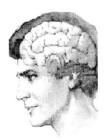

MALE
In the man the two
sex chromosomes are
XY.

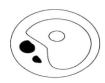

The ovum of the woman, however,
contains only X chromosomes

X   Y

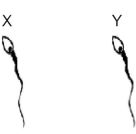

Some sperm of the man contain X
chromosomes; others contain Y
chromosomes.

With this in mind, many couples worldwide who have several children of the same
sex, have used this information to time their marital relations accordingly to
conceive a girl or a boy.

Studies indicate that the sperm with Y
chromosome swim faster, but survive only 24
hours, while the sperm with X chromosome swim
more slowly, but survive approximately two to
three days.

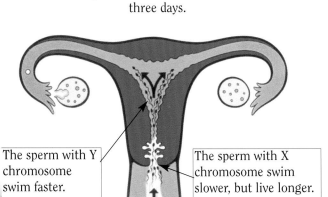

The sperm with Y
chromosome
swim faster.

The sperm with X
chromosome swim
slower, but live longer.

Infertile Days   **Fertile Days**

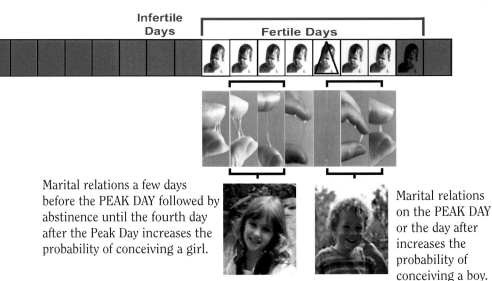

Marital relations a few days
before the PEAK DAY followed by
abstinence until the fourth day
after the Peak Day increases the
probability of conceiving a girl.

Marital relations
on the PEAK DAY
or the day after
increases the
probability of
conceiving a boy.

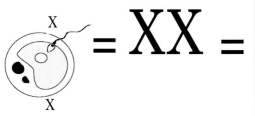 = XX =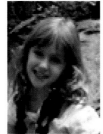

When the X type sperm unites with the ovum of the wife, the baby is a girl.

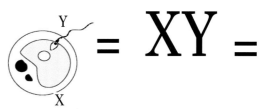 = XY =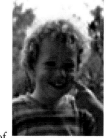

When the Y type sperm unites with the ovum of the wife, the baby is a boy

According to Dr. Evelyn Billings, "The scientific evidence on this is controversial. Some users say that marital relations early in the development of fertile type mucus with no other coitus during that cycle, tends to result in a girl; while marital relations confined to the day of the Peak fertility tends to result in a boy. A study in Nigeria appears to confirm this tendency. This study was based on the theory that a single act of marital relations at the Peak would result in a boy; while marital relations when the mucus changed from sticky and became slippery before the Peak, with no further marital relations until after the fertile phase was over, would result in a girl."[1]

Infertile Days

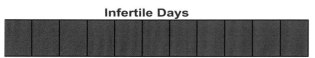

According to the study coordinator, Dr. (Sr.) Leonie McSweeney:
"Success in pre-selection of a boy was achieved by 310 couples. Failure in pre-selection of a boy occurred in four couples. Success in pre-selection of a girl was achieved in 90 couples. Failure in pre-selection of a girl occurred in two couples. Others who have tried to use the method to pre-select the sex of a child have generally achieved a lower success rate. Pre-determination of the sex of a baby is never likely to be 100 percent reliable."[2]

Additionally, another study by Dr. (Sr.) Leonie McSweeney: stated: "Hormonal studies have shown that in a high percentage of cases, ovulation takes place within 24-48 hours of the Peak symptom. Therefore, if marital relations take place on the Peak day and are repeated the next day and if the ovum is already waiting or is released soon after marital relations, the Y-bearing sperm is much more likely to fertilize the ovum resulting in the conception of a male child. But if marital relations take place before the Peak symptom and the ovum for that cycle does not arrive for 24 hours, then it would seem likely that a female child would be conceived."[3] A new study by Dr. (Sr.) Leonie McSweeney published in the African Journal of Reproductive Health, March 2011, gives additional and more detailed data on the subject.

1. Dr. Evelyn Billings and Anne Westmore, *The Billings Method, Controlling fertility without drugs or devices*, Life Cycle Books, 2000, p. 70-71.
2. McSweeney, Dr. Sr. Leonie, "A Prospective Study of Sex Preselection in Ondo, Nigeria, using the Billings Ovulation Method of Natural Family Planning", *Bulletin of the Natural Family Planning Council of Victoria*, Vol. 20, No. 4, p. 9-16, 1993.
3. McSweeney, Dr. Sr. Leonie, "Successful Sex Pre-selection using Natural Family Planning", *African Journal of Reproductive Health*, March 2011; 15(1), p. 79-83.

V.

Guidelines to Postpone Pregnancy

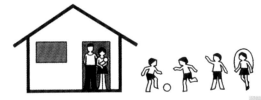

Variation between Peak Day and Menstruation

Peak Day

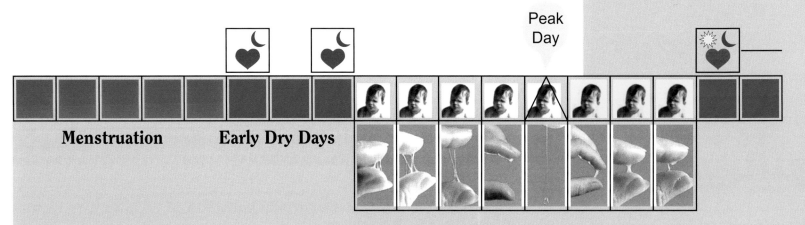

Menstruation   Early Dry Days

Early Days of the Cycle - The Preovulatory Phase

The early days of the cycle extend from the beginning of menstruation to the PEAK DAY. In these days of the cycle there is usually a time of infertility when the reproductive hormones are at a low level. This infertile time manifests itself in the woman by a sensation of dryness at the vulva. Any change from this pattern indicates rising levels of hormones and possible fertility. The Early Day Rules are applied to postpone pregnancy during this phase of the cycle. These rules are designed to enable the woman to recognize the beginning of the fertile phase and to identify the PEAK DAY. In the early days of the cycle, when the woman feels dry, marital relations are open to the couple only in the evening so that the return to dryness can be confirmed during the day. Marital relations on alternate evenings are available to the spouses. This allows for accurate observation so that seminal fluid and vaginal secretions do not obscure the recognition of cervical mucus. See pages 68-70.

The Late Days of the Cycle - The Post-Peak Phase

The late days of the cycle extend from the PEAK DAY symptom (the last day that the mucus is wet and slippery) to the next menstruation.

When learning the Ovulation Method, abstinence is recommended for 2 to 4 weeks in order for the woman to learn to identify her individual fertile mucus pattern.

The days between the Peak Day and Menstruation vary between 10 to 16 days. If it is less than 10 days, it was an anovulatory cycle. If it is more than 16 days, she may be pregnant.

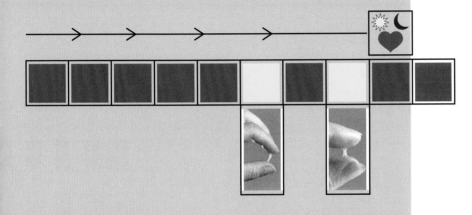

The PEAK DAY indicates that ovulation is near or has just taken place. The PEAK DAY is recognized the day after it occurs by the change to dryness or to sticky type mucus. Please see page 60.

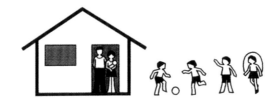

IF, on the other hand, <u>YOU NEED TO SPACE YOUR PREGNANCIES, OR NOT BECOME PREGNANT AT ALL</u>, you must adhere to the following Rules:

There are three Early Day Rules:
(The early days of the cycle extend from the beginning of menstruation to the PEAK DAY).

AVOID MARITAL RELATIONS ON THE DAYS OF MENSTRUAL BLEEDING.
The reason for this is that the brain may send the signal to the ovaries earlier than usual and blood may mask the mucus, making it difficult for the woman to know that her time of fertility has started. Additionally, there is medical support for abstinence during menstruation; there is evidence that women who engage in marital relations during menstruation increase their risk of endometriosis.*

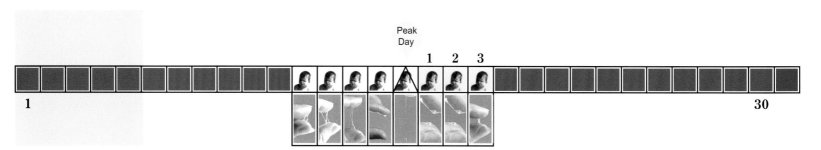

Peak Day
1 2 3
1
30

---

* Filer, Robert and Wu Chung, "Coitus During Menses: Its effect on endometriosis & Pelvic Inflammatory disease" Journal of Reproductive Medicine, November, 1989; p. 887-890.

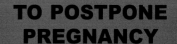

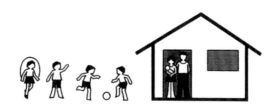

2 DURING THE EARLY DRY DAYS, MARITAL RELATIONS ARE OPEN TO THE COUPLE ONLY EVERY OTHER EVENING, <u>NOT</u> ON TWO CONSECUTIVE EVENINGS.

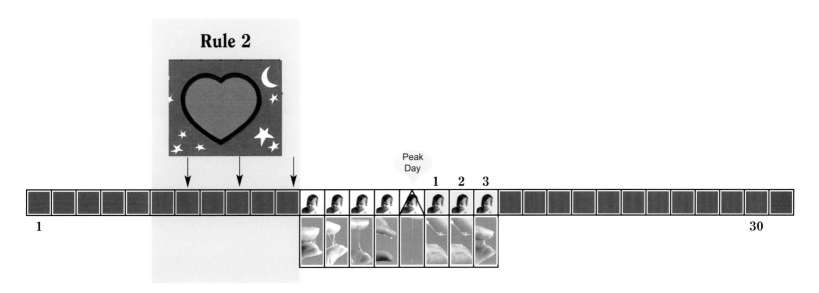

The reason for this Rule is to observe throughout the day for any change from dryness, and to ensure that seminal fluid will not mask the beginning of the fertile phase.

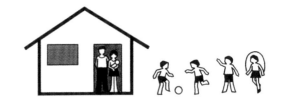

AVOID MARITAL RELATIONS DURING THE DAYS OF ANY CHANGE FROM DRYNESS TO MUCUS, WETNESS OR BLEEDING PLUS THE FOLLOWING THREE FULL DAYS.

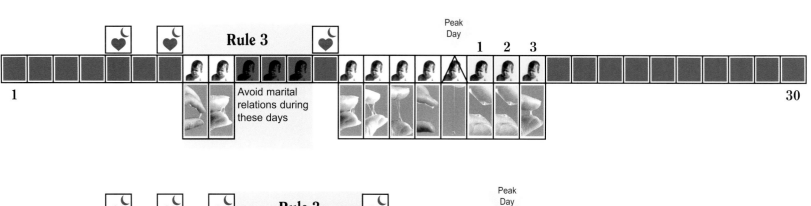

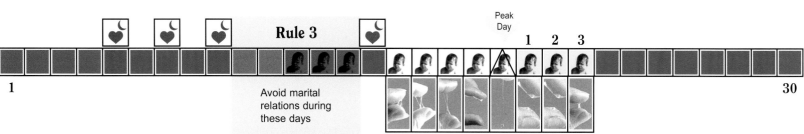

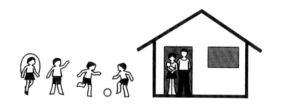

The Peak Day Rule:

WHEN THE PEAK DAY IS ESTABLISHED <u>WITH CERTAINTY</u>, MARITAL RELATIONS ARE OPEN TO THE COUPLE FROM THE MORNING OF THE FOURTH DAY AFTER THE PEAK UNTIL THE NEXT MENSTRUATION BEGINS.

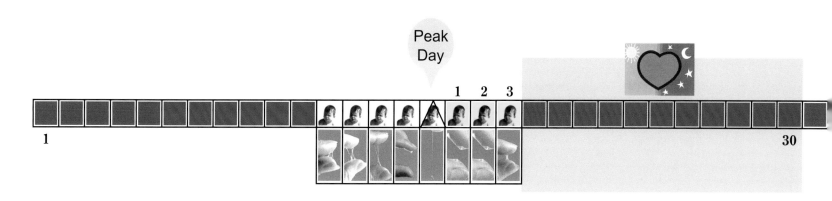

........from this fourth day on until menstruation begins, pregnancy is not possible and there are no restrictions on marital relations.

- Average Cycle

Peak Day

 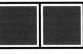 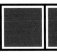

During the days of menstruation apply Rule 1: *"Avoid marital relations on the days of menstrual bleeding."* There is medical support for abstinence during menstruation. The incidence of endometriosis is significantly higher in women who have marital relations during their menstrual period. Endometriosis increases probability of infertility as a result of the inflammatory process associated with it.*

Dry days. These are the infertile days of her cycle. She applied Rule 2: *"During the Early Dry Days, marital relations are open to the couple only every other evening, <u>not</u> on two consecutive evenings."*

On the ninth day she observed a cloudy, sticky mucus, this means the fertile phase had begun. To postpone pregnancy abstinence is necessary from this day on.

The woman observed the mucus was becoming progressively clearer and more elastic with a wet, slippery sensation. Abstinence continued during the days of mucus with fertile characteristics, which is usually accompanied by a sensation of wetness.

This day she observed a change to cloudy, sticky mucus; this was her indication to mark the PEAK DAY which was the previous day. Once the Peak Day was identified with certainty, the couple applied the Peak Day Rule and abstained for three full days.

* Filer, Robert and Wu Chung, "Coitus During Menses: Its effect on endometriosis & Pelvic Inflammatory disease" Journal of Reproductive Medicine, November, 1989; p. 887-890.

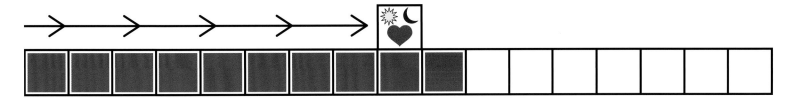

The remaining days were open to the couple for marital relations at any time, day or night, until the next menstruation.

Special Considerations
— If a woman is uncertain that she has identified the PEAK DAY, she should continue to consider herself in the early days of the cycle to which the Early Day Rules apply. Please see pages 68-71.
— If menstruation does not occur within 16 days after the PEAK DAY symptom, it is likely that the PEAK DAY was incorrectly identified. The woman should then apply the Early Day Rules so that the fertile phase and the true PEAK DAY can be recognized when it occurs.
— Bleeding which is not preceded by the PEAK DAY, 10 to 16 days earlier, may not be a true menstruation. Please see pages 78-79. In such circumstances the couple should abstain for 3 full days following the bleeding and continue to apply the Early Day Rules until the PEAK DAY is identified.

Short Cycle

Short cycles are normal for some women. In a short cycle a woman may notice the mucus beginning earlier, even overlapping with menstruation or perhaps changing rapidly to the Peak. Mucus may even begin during the days of menstrual bleeding. However, at any time in her life, a woman may have a variation in cycle length.

Following is an example of a woman's short cycle.

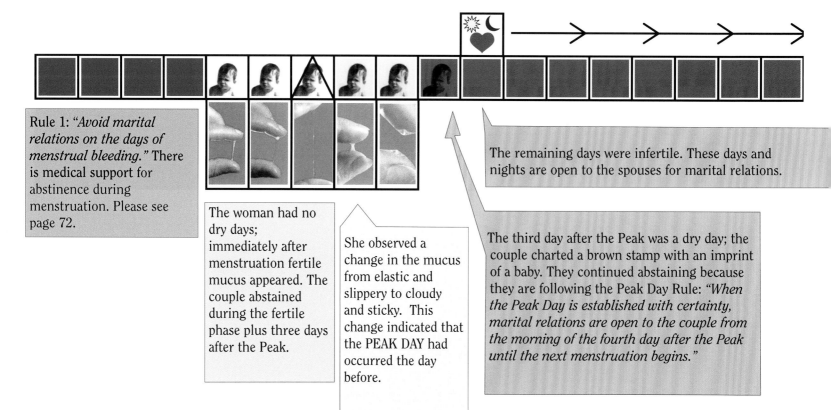

Rule 1: *"Avoid marital relations on the days of menstrual bleeding."* There is medical support for abstinence during menstruation. Please see page 72.

The woman had no dry days; immediately after menstruation fertile mucus appeared. The couple abstained during the fertile phase plus three days after the Peak.

She observed a change in the mucus from elastic and slippery to cloudy and sticky. This change indicated that the PEAK DAY had occurred the day before.

The remaining days were infertile. These days and nights are open to the spouses for marital relations.

The third day after the Peak was a dry day; the couple charted a brown stamp with an imprint of a baby. They continued abstaining because they are following the Peak Day Rule: *"When the Peak Day is established with certainty, marital relations are open to the couple from the morning of the fourth day after the Peak until the next menstruation begins."*

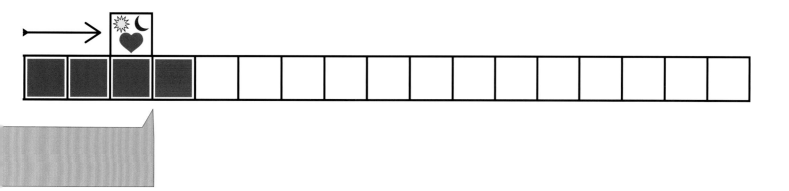

Special Considerations
— If a woman is uncertain that she has identified the PEAK DAY, she should continue to consider herself in the early days of the cycle to which the Early Day Rules apply. Please see pages 68-71.
— If menstruation does not occur within 16 days after the PEAK DAY symptom, it is likely that the PEAK DAY was incorrectly identified. The woman should then apply the Early Day Rules so that the fertile phase and the true PEAK DAY can be recognized when it occurs.
— Bleeding which is not preceded by the PEAK DAY, 10 to 16 days earlier, may not be a true menstruation. Please see pages 78-79. In such circumstances the couple should abstain for 3 full days following the bleeding and continue to apply the Early Day Rules until the PEAK DAY is identified.

Long Cycle

The long cycle is another variation of cycle length. Long cycles are normal for some women and in other women may be the result of stress, illness, medication or poor nutrition that delays ovulation. An extended period of dryness after menstruation or occasional mucus patches before the fertile phase begins, is not unusual in this type of cycle.

This is an example of a woman's long cycle who suffered stress after the death of her father. The fertile phase had begun but was temporarily suspended.

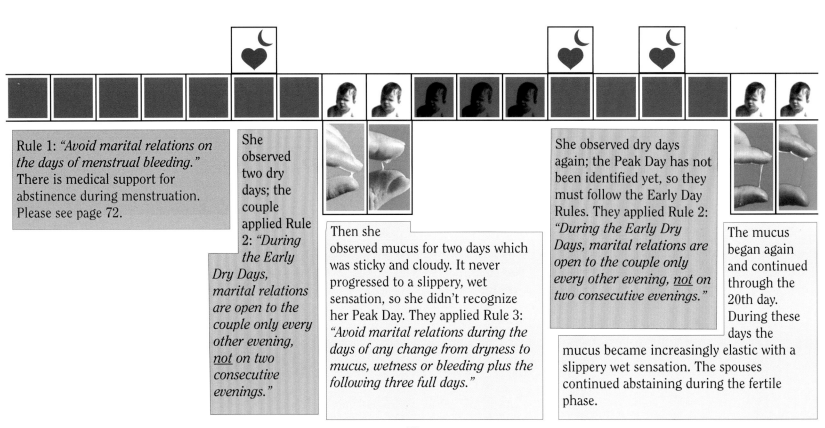

Rule 1: *"Avoid marital relations on the days of menstrual bleeding."* There is medical support for abstinence during menstruation. Please see page 72.

She observed two dry days; the couple applied Rule 2: *"During the Early Dry Days, marital relations are open to the couple only every other evening, not on two consecutive evenings."*

Then she observed mucus for two days which was sticky and cloudy. It never progressed to a slippery, wet sensation, so she didn't recognize her Peak Day. They applied Rule 3: *"Avoid marital relations during the days of any change from dryness to mucus, wetness or bleeding plus the following three full days."*

She observed dry days again; the Peak Day has not been identified yet, so they must follow the Early Day Rules. They applied Rule 2: *"During the Early Dry Days, marital relations are open to the couple only every other evening, not on two consecutive evenings."*

The mucus began again and continued through the 20th day. During these days the mucus became increasingly elastic with a slippery wet sensation. The spouses continued abstaining during the fertile phase.

Some women under special circumstances may experience very long cycles (i.e., those coming off the pill and other artificial methods, during stress, being overweight, underweight, during pre-menopause...). They may experience cycles longer than 35 days or may not ovulate at all for months, depending on the individual woman and the suppression of ovulation occasioned by the different circumstances. In these cases there are specific guidelines designed to enable the woman to recognize the return of fertility by the appearance of cervical mucus and the identification of the Peak. These rules are under "Guidelines to postpone pregnancy while Breastfeeding and Very long cycles," on pages 84-89. To postpone pregnancy during special circumstances see pages 96-103.

Important: If a woman is uncertain that she has identified the PEAK DAY, she should continue to consider herself in the early days of the cycle to which the Early Day Rules apply.

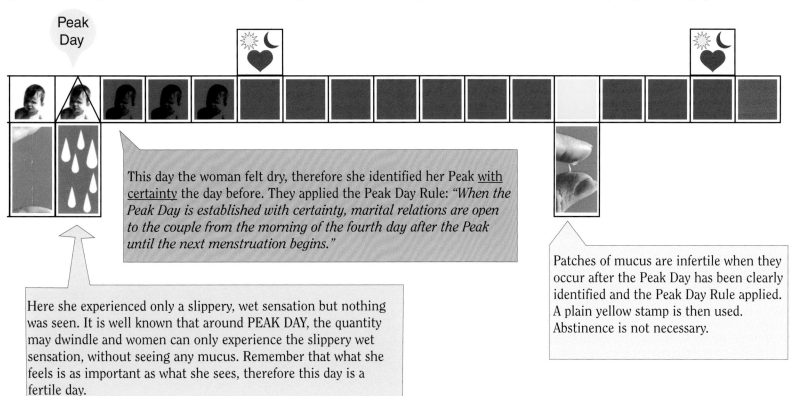

Peak
Day

This day the woman felt dry, therefore she identified her Peak <u>with certainty</u> the day before. They applied the Peak Day Rule: *"When the Peak Day is established with certainty, marital relations are open to the couple from the morning of the fourth day after the Peak until the next menstruation begins."*

Here she experienced only a slippery, wet sensation but nothing was seen. It is well known that around PEAK DAY, the quantity may dwindle and women can only experience the slippery wet sensation, without seeing any mucus. Remember that what she feels is as important as what she sees, therefore this day is a fertile day.

Patches of mucus are infertile when they occur after the Peak Day has been clearly identified and the Peak Day Rule applied. A plain yellow stamp is then used. Abstinence is not necessary.

Anovulatory Cycle

Any women may experience a cycle in which there is no ovulation. Anovulatory cycles may be caused by illness, medication, stress, a nutritional deficiency, overweight, underweight or other factors. This is an example of a woman's anovulatory cycle.

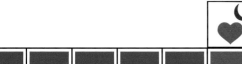

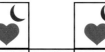

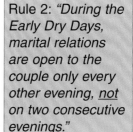

Rule 1: *"Avoid marital relations on the days of menstrual bleeding."* There is medical support for abstinence during menstruation. Please see page 72.

She had three dry days; the spouses applied Rule 2: *"During the Early Dry Days, marital relations are open to the couple only every other evening, not on two consecutive evenings."*

She observed a day of mucus followed by 6 dry days; they applied Rule 3: *"Avoid marital relations during the days of any change from dryness to mucus, wetness or bleeding plus the following three full days."*
The mucus was cloudy and sticky; she did not recognize a normal pattern of fertility and therefore continued following the Early Day Rules.

Rule 2: *"During the Early Dry Days, marital relations are open to the couple only every other evening, not on two consecutive evenings."*

She again observed a patch of mucus with infertile characteristics. They applied Rule 3 and abstained during the days of mucus and the following three complete dry days.

The couple followed the Early Day Rules throughout the cycle. Each time there was a change **from dryness, the** couple abstained through the days of change (mucus or bleeding) and for **the three** days which followed the change back to **dryness. Then,** the evening of every other dry day was open to the couple for marital relations.

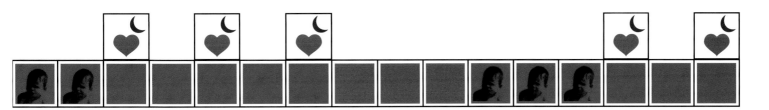

Important:
There are several factors that are important to understand in an anovulatory cycle. It is identified in retrospect by the following characteristic elements:
a) The absence of a fertile pattern of mucus.
b) The absence of the Peak symptom.

This bleeding was not a true menstruation. As ovulation has not occurred (there was no Peak Day). The bleed may also disguise signs of fertility which accompany ovulation. It is for this reason that the couple should avoid marital relations during the bleed until dryness has returned for three days. They applied Rule 3: *"Avoid marital relations during the days of any change from dryness to mucus, wetness or bleeding plus the following three full days."*

The couple then should continue to consider themselves in the early days of the cycle, applying the Early Day Rules until the Peak is identified.

VI.

Breastfeeding

During breastfeeding, the brain temporarily stops the ovaries' activities in order to protect the body's ability to provide nourishment to the baby. Breastfeeding is a natural and ideal way of feeding the baby. It helps the baby develop better physically and emotionally. The mother's defenses against infection are passed on to the baby through her milk. When a woman is breastfeeding, she can learn to recognize a pattern of infertility which indicates inactivity of the ovaries. This will either be a feeling of constant dryness or an unchanging discharge, day after day after day (Fig. 50). This type of discharge is quite different from the mucus seen when a woman is ovulating normally, and so we will mark it on the chart with a different color stamp -- YELLOW.

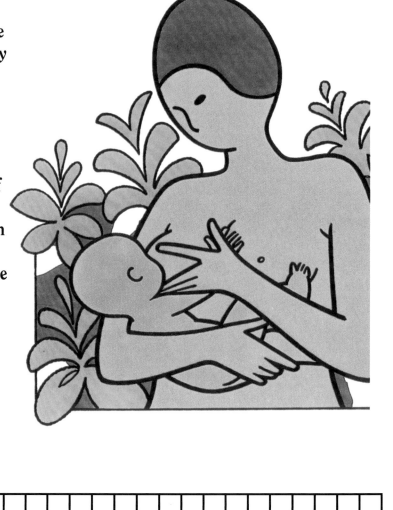

Fig. 50

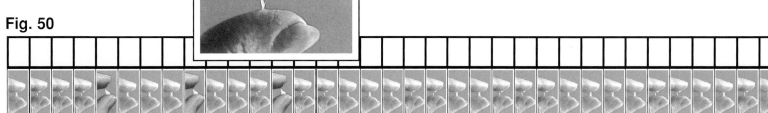

But when will the wet, slippery mucus return to tell us the clock has started up again? Apparently, nature prefers to set things in motion gradually -- with a series of little spurts and starts. It is generally only when the baby no longer obtains its nourishment solely from the mother's breast that the brain starts the mechanism up again. Then the pituitary sends the signal to the ovaries to begin the maturing of the follicle and the release of the ovum (Fig. 51).

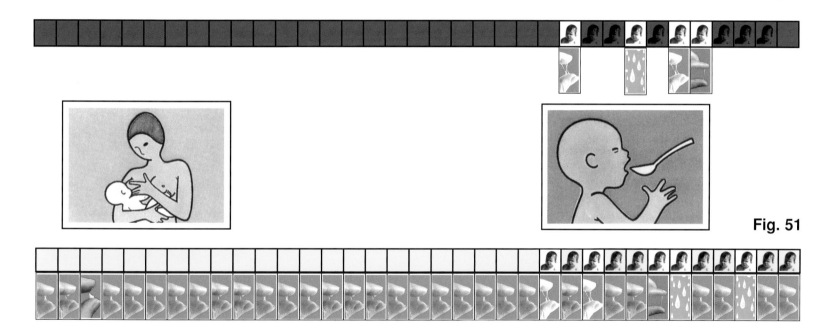

Fig. 51

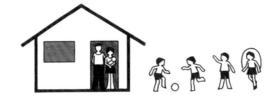

What should the couple do when a woman has very long cycles or is breastfeeding?

During these times, which may last weeks or even months, the woman knows that she is NOT FERTILE, either because of dryness or because of the constant presence of an unchanging vaginal discharge, which remains the same day after day after day. This discharge is quite different from the mucus seen when a woman is ovulating normally, and must be observed for two weeks without change before it is considered infertile, or what we call the Basic Infertile Pattern (B.I.P.) of discharge.

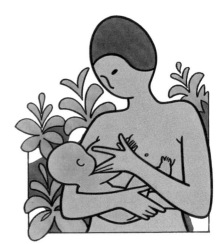

BASIC INFERTILE PATTERN (B.I.P.)

By careful observation a woman can learn to recognize her time of infertility, which is manifested by either a sensation at the vulva of dryness or by an unchanging discharge present at the vulva for two weeks; the way a woman manifests her infertility is called: Basic Infertile Pattern (B.I.P.). Any change from this pattern is the indication that the return of fertility is approaching. This understanding is especially important in women with very long cycles (longer than 35 days) such as: breastfeeding mothers, coming off artificial methods, in times of stress, pre-menopause, and some women with overweight or underweight issues, or anyone taking daily prescription medication.

Charting After Childbirth

A woman begins charting after childbirth when blood loss (lochia) begins to stop, usually around three weeks after the birth. If the mother is nursing her baby, she will feel constantly dry or will have an unchanging milky type discharge. Abstinence is recommended until her B.I.P. is established, which takes two weeks (please see page 86). Then the Early Day Rules are applied to postpone pregnancy. These rules are designed to enable the woman to recognize the return of fertility, the beginning of the fertile phase and the identification of the Peak.

The guidelines to postpone pregnancy while breastfeeding and in women with very long cycles are on pages 86-89.

IMPORTANT:

During breastfeeding or very long cycles, any bleeding that occurs before identifying the PEAK DAY (and confirmed by menstrual bleeding 10 to 16 days after) is considered possibly fertile and the couple should abstain during the days of bleeding plus the following three full days. When the woman identifies with certainty her PEAK DAY and it is confirmed by menstruation 10 to 16 days after, she can consider that she has returned to her regular cycles.

BREASTFEEDING

Mothers who are fully breastfeeding their babies may not ovulate or menstruate for several months. Fully breastfeeding means that the baby is dependent entirely on the breast for nutrition, with no supplementary formula or the use of pacifiers. Suckling stimulates the production of a hormone (prolactin) that suppresses ovulation, thus delaying the woman's return to fertility. Suckling frequently, on demand, and using the breast as a pacifier or comforter usually delays the onset of ovulation. Once the need for milk diminishes, as when supplemental food is added or the baby is weaned, this hormone is decreased and the woman begins to return to fertility.

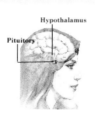

Prolactin inhibits ovulation

As long as mother is nursing baby, Prolactin levels will remain high and will suppress FSH and LH from starting fertile phase.

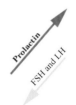

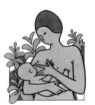

Prolactin produces milk

The more the baby suckles the longer ovulation is inhibited

Common discharge among breastfeeding mothers: (BIP of discharge)

A breastfeeding mother or a woman with very long cycles recognizes her time of infertility by either a sensation at the vulva of dryness or by an unchanging discharge present at the vulva. This time of infertility is called: the *Basic Infertile Pattern* (B.I.P.). A woman needs to establish her B.I.P. by observing her pattern, which does not change in quantity, quality or sensation for two weeks. Any change from this pattern is the indication that the return of fertility is approaching.

- Basic Infertile Pattern of Dryness

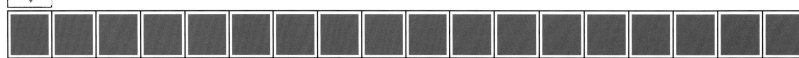

When a woman observes her infertility as dryness, we say that she has a *Basic Infertile Pattern of Dryness.* This is an example of a woman who fully breastfed her baby. When the lochia ceased, she charted dryness. She observed no mucus, spotting or bleeding and did not experience a change from the sensation of dryness. Once the B.I.P. of dryness was identified, the couple applied the Early Day Rules to postpone pregnancy. Marital relations were open

- Basic Infertile Pattern of Discharge

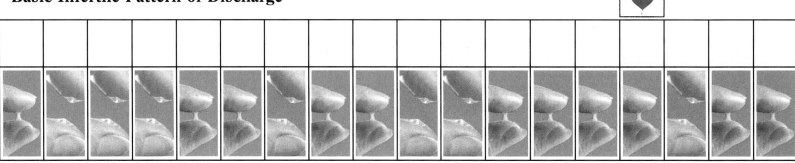

Sometimes a woman observes her infertility as a continuous discharge, which is a *Basic Infertile Pattern of Discharge.* This type of secretion has no substance, so when it dries it leaves no residue, unlike slippery mucus, which has substance and may stretch. This example shows a woman who fully breastfed her baby and experienced an unchanging discharge.

The couple abstained for two weeks while the woman charted a constant mucus discharge that remained the same day after day after day. Once she observed that it did not change in quality, quantity or sensation for two weeks, the B.I.P. of discharge was established. From that point, the couple applied the Early Day Rules to postpone pregnancy.

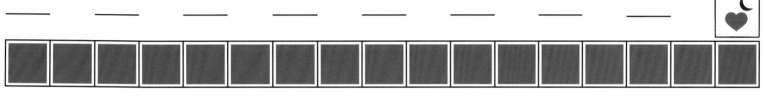

to the couple on the evening of every other dry day. They should abstain on days of any change plus the following three dry days.

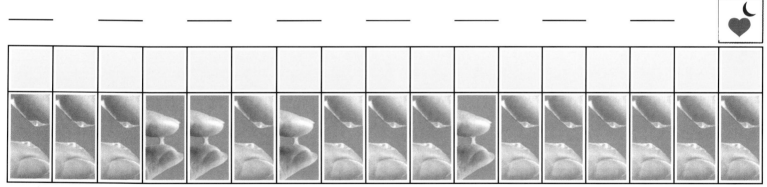

Marital relations were open to the couple on the evening of every other day of unchanging discharge.

Some women experience a pattern of unchanging discharge with intermittent dry days. Once this pattern has been observed for two weeks, and confirmed by the instructor, it is considered a B.I.P. The couple then applies the Early Day Rules to postpone pregnancy. Marital relations are open to the couple on the evening of every other day of this combined B.I.P. until any change occurs.

Any change in the mucus discharge such as an increase in the amount, a change in the sensation it produces, the development of stretchiness or greater clarity, or the addition of blood which would tinge the discharge red, pink or yellow, indicates possible fertility. The couple would then avoid marital relations through the days of change plus the three full days that follow the change back to the same unchanging discharge (or to dryness).

Rules to postpone pregnancy while breastfeeding and during very long cycles.

> **MARITAL RELATIONS ARE OPEN TO THE COUPLE ONLY EVERY OTHER EVENING, <u>NOT</u> ON TWO CONSECUTIVE EVENINGS, AFTER OBSERVING THROUGHOUT THE DAY FOR ANY CHANGE FROM THESE PATTERNS.**
>
> See page 69 for additional information.

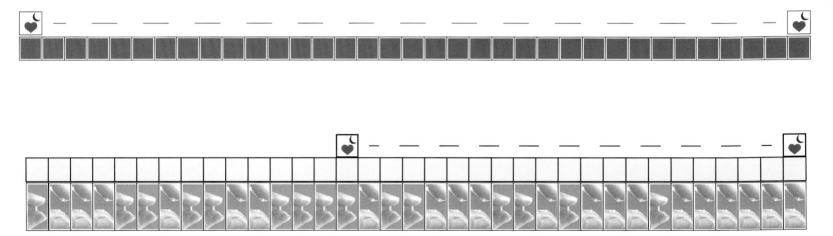

AVOID MARITAL RELATIONS ALTOGETHER WHEN THERE IS A CHANGE* FROM DRYNESS UNTIL THE FOURTH EVENING AFTER THE SAME PATTERN OF INFERTILITY RETURNS... and continue to apply the Early Day Rules.

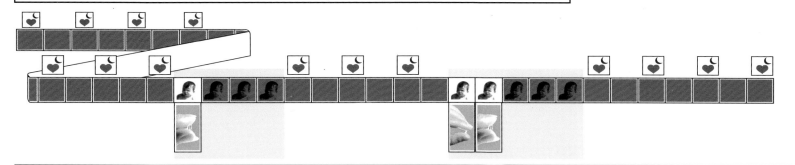

AVOID MARITAL RELATIONS ALTOGETHER WHEN THERE IS A CHANGE* FROM THE UNCHANGING DISCHARGE UNTIL THE FOURTH EVENING AFTER THE SAME PATTERN OF INFERTILITY RETURNS... and continue to apply the Early Day Rules.

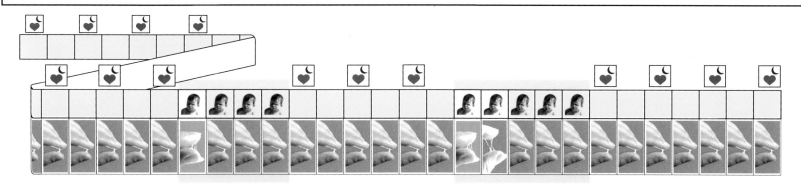

*NOTE: A change can be in the appearance of mucus; a wet or slippery sensation; a change in the amount of the discharge; or a change in its color or consistency.

Patches of mucus may appear at any time during breastfeeding and, in particular, when nursing is decreasing. This example shows a woman who had already established a Basic Infertile Pattern (B.I.P.) of dryness and experienced mucus patches when nursing was decreased on two occasions, when the mother and then the baby were ill. The mucus patches disappeared when the number of feedings returned to normal. The couple followed the Early Day Rules throughout this time.

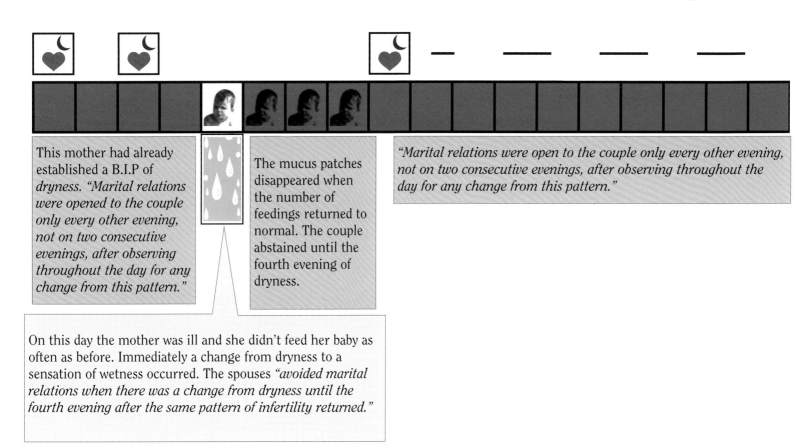

This mother had already established a B.I.P of *dryness*. *"Marital relations were opened to the couple only every other evening, not on two consecutive evenings, after observing throughout the day for any change from this pattern."*

The mucus patches disappeared when the number of feedings returned to normal. The couple abstained until the fourth evening of dryness.

"Marital relations were open to the couple only every other evening, not on two consecutive evenings, after observing throughout the day for any change from this pattern."

On this day the mother was ill and she didn't feed her baby as often as before. Immediately a change from dryness to a sensation of wetness occurred. The spouses *"avoided marital relations when there was a change from dryness until the fourth evening after the same pattern of infertility returned."*

When there was a change from the B.I.P. of dryness, the couple abstained the days of change and for the three full days that followed the change back to the B.I.P. (i.e., the evening of the fourth day was available).

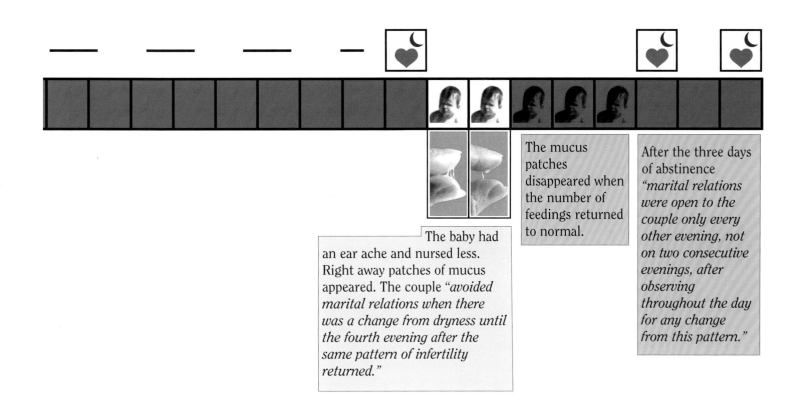

The baby had an ear ache and nursed less. Right away patches of mucus appeared. The couple *"avoided marital relations when there was a change from dryness until the fourth evening after the same pattern of infertility returned."*

The mucus patches disappeared when the number of feedings returned to normal.

After the three days of abstinence *"marital relations were open to the couple only every other evening, not on two consecutive evenings, after observing throughout the day for any change from this pattern."*

The return of fertility may be prompted by a reduced number of feedings as the baby is given additional solid foods or other fluids. Fertility may also closely follow any ill health the mother or child experiences, which causes a decrease in breastfeeding. If weaning is gradual, there may be several patches of mucus before ovulation occurs.

Sometimes a slippery sensation, without any obvious stretchy mucus, is the only sign of fertility, due to the decreased level of prolactin (the hormone that produces the milk for the baby). Thus the first ovulation may not be preceded by abundant, clear, stretchy mucus but only a wet, slippery sensation. This is an example of a woman's chart during weaning.

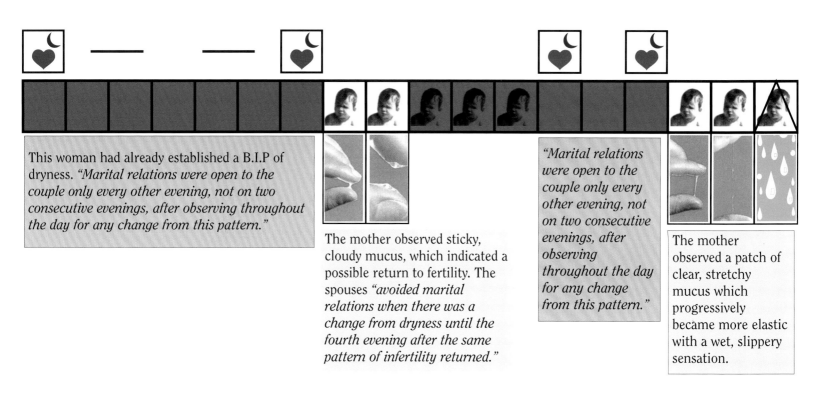

This woman had already established a B.I.P of dryness. *"Marital relations were open to the couple only every other evening, not on two consecutive evenings, after observing throughout the day for any change from this pattern."*

The mother observed sticky, cloudy mucus, which indicated a possible return to fertility. The spouses *"avoided marital relations when there was a change from dryness until the fourth evening after the same pattern of infertility returned."*

"Marital relations were open to the couple only every other evening, not on two consecutive evenings, after observing throughout the day for any change from this pattern."

The mother observed a patch of clear, stretchy mucus which progressively became more elastic with a wet, slippery sensation.

It is **important** to understand that weaning triggers hormonal changes that begin the return of fertility. Frequent patches of mucus can occur at this time. Abstinence for a few weeks may be helpful to the mother until she identifies the PEAK DAY. A breastfeeding mother who is carefully observing her mucus patches will be warned of the return of fertility well in advance.

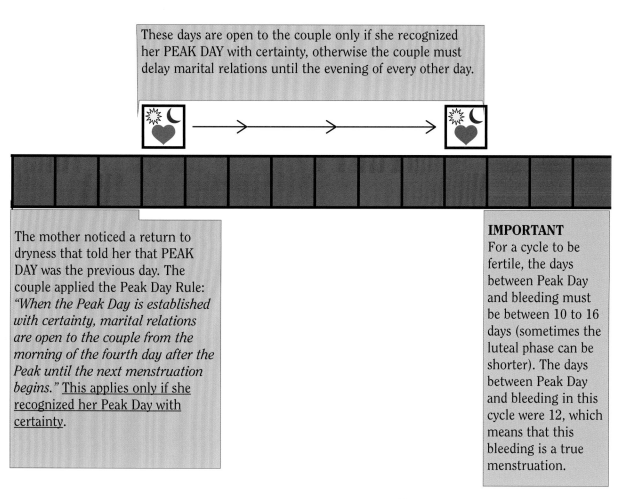

These days are open to the couple only if she recognized her PEAK DAY with certainty, otherwise the couple must delay marital relations until the evening of every other day.

The mother noticed a return to dryness that told her that PEAK DAY was the previous day. The couple applied the Peak Day Rule: *"When the Peak Day is established with certainty, marital relations are open to the couple from the morning of the fourth day after the Peak until the next menstruation begins."* This applies only if she recognized her Peak Day with certainty.

IMPORTANT
For a cycle to be fertile, the days between Peak Day and bleeding must be between 10 to 16 days (sometimes the luteal phase can be shorter). The days between Peak Day and bleeding in this cycle were 12, which means that this bleeding is a true menstruation.

VII.

Postponing Pregnancy: Special Circumstances

These varieties of charts are found in special circumstances such as: STRESS, DISCONTINUED USE OF THE PILL, IMPLANT, *DEPO-PROVERA*, THE PATCH or INTRAUTERINE DEVICES and DURING PREMENOPAUSE.

Any mucus secretion observed during the early days of a cycle is considered possibly fertile. In special circumstances such as stress, coming off artificial methods and during pre-menopause, the ovaries are working in spurts trying to ovulate, but the process is not always completed. It may be interrupted due to having affected the normal function of the ovaries, which suppressed the necessary elevation of hormones for ovulation to occur. When the ovaries are trying to return to normal, hormonal levels increase and patches of mucus appear that eventually lead to ovulation.

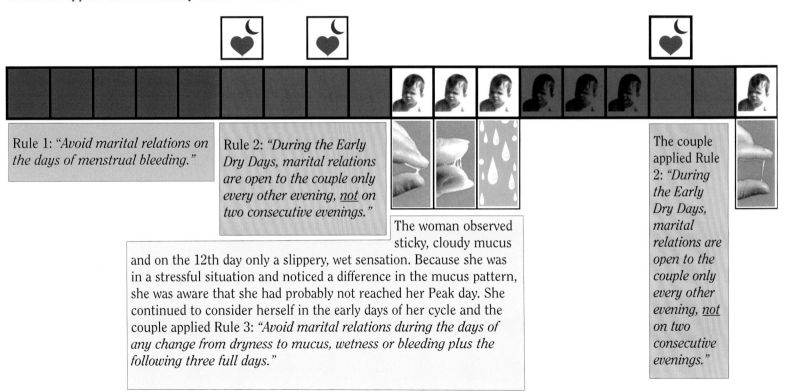

Rule 1: *"Avoid marital relations on the days of menstrual bleeding."*

Rule 2: *"During the Early Dry Days, marital relations are open to the couple only every other evening, not on two consecutive evenings."*

The woman observed sticky, cloudy mucus and on the 12th day only a slippery, wet sensation. Because she was in a stressful situation and noticed a difference in the mucus pattern, she was aware that she had probably not reached her Peak day. She continued to consider herself in the early days of her cycle and the couple applied Rule 3: *"Avoid marital relations during the days of any change from dryness to mucus, wetness or bleeding plus the following three full days."*

The couple applied Rule 2: *"During the Early Dry Days, marital relations are open to the couple only every other evening, not on two consecutive evenings."*

The days between PEAK DAY and bleeding were 13. Therefore this bleeding is a true menstruation and she recognized her Peak Day correctly.

Peak Day

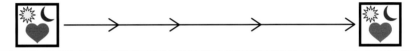

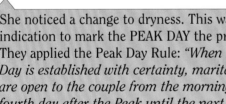

She noticed a change to dryness. This was her indication to mark the PEAK DAY the previous day. They applied the Peak Day Rule: *"When the Peak Day is established with certainty, marital relations are open to the couple from the morning of the fourth day after the Peak until the next menstruation begins."*

The woman observed stretchy, slippery mucus and felt the sensation of wetness, which she identified as the return of her mucus pattern.

Special Considerations:

— If a woman is uncertain that she has identified the PEAK DAY, she should continue to consider herself in the early days of the cycle to which the Early Day Rules apply.

— If menstruation does not occur within 16 days after the PEAK DAY symptom, it is likely that the PEAK DAY was incorrectly identified. The woman should then apply the Early Day Rules so that the fertile phase and the true PEAK DAY can be recognized when they occur.

All mucus observed in the early days of a cycle is considered possibly fertile. Some women may experience a constant discharge before the fertile phase begins. Constant discharge means a secretion with no change in amount, sensation, consistency or color that remains the same day after day before the fertile phase begins. This is due to low circulatory levels of estrogen. When she observes an increase in the amount of mucus, a change in the sensation, the development of stretchiness or greater transparency, or the addition of blood which tinges the discharge red, pink or yellow, it is an indication of possible fertility. Some women manifest their infertility with an unchanging discharge. To consider this discharge as infertile, they must accomplish the following requirements:

- The woman must be able to recognize with certainty the difference between the constant secretion she observes after menstruation to any change in amount, color, consistency or a slippery wet sensation.

-The woman consistently observed mucus with basically no change from the end of menstruation to the beginning of the fertile phase during 3 consecutive cycles and this was confirmed by her instructor.

In women with very long cycles with continuous discharge, the secretion must remain constant and unchanged for fourteen consecutive days, please see pages 76-77. This constant discharge is called the Basic Infertile Pattern of Discharge (B.I.P. of Discharge). Any change from this pattern is the indication that the return of fertility is approaching.

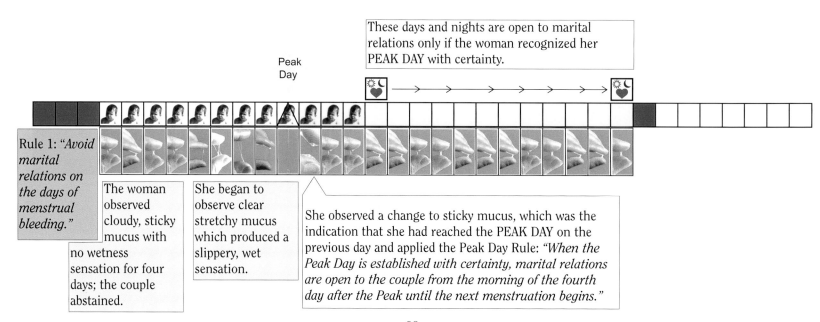

Peak
Day

These days and nights are open to marital relations only if the woman recognized her PEAK DAY with certainty.

Rule 1: *"Avoid marital relations on the days of menstrual bleeding."*

The woman observed cloudy, sticky mucus with no wetness sensation for four days; the couple abstained.

She began to observe clear stretchy mucus which produced a slippery, wet sensation.

She observed a change to sticky mucus, which was the indication that she had reached the PEAK DAY on the previous day and applied the Peak Day Rule: *"When the Peak Day is established with certainty, marital relations are open to the couple from the morning of the fourth day after the Peak until the next menstruation begins."*

The woman observed basically the same pattern of unchanging discharge during the following 2 cycles.

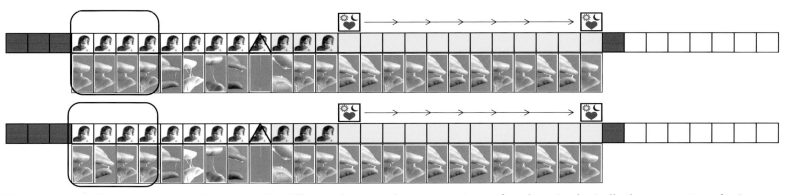

The woman was able to recognize with certainty the difference between the two secretions. After observing basically the same pattern for 3 consecutive cycles and confirmed by an instructor, the couple used the plain yellow stamps and followed the Early Day Rules:

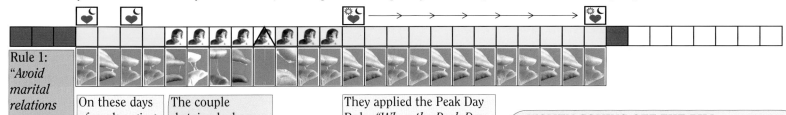

Rule 1: *"Avoid marital relations on the days of menstrual bleeding."*

On these days of unchanging discharge the couple applied Rule 2: *"During the Early Dry Days, marital relations are open to the couple only every other evening, not on two consecutive evenings."*

The couple abstained when she observed a change from her B.I.P. of Discharge that indicated to her the beginning of the fertile phase.

They applied the Peak Day Rule: *"When the Peak Day is recognized with certainty, marital relations are open to the couple from the morning of the fourth day after the Peak until the next menstruation begins."*

WOMEN COMING OFF THE PILL
Women coming off the pill often experience a constant mucus secretion, which usually slowly disappears. The return of ovulation (and thus the Peak Day) may occur within a few weeks. However, depending on the individual woman and the suppression of ovarian function caused by the Pill and the dosage used, ovulation may not occur for several months. Strong ovarian pain may accompany her first ovulation after discontinuation of the pill. Women discontinuing the pill should abstain from marital relations during the first month of charting to make careful observations of the pattern of fertility or infertility. The couple must follow the Early Day Rules until she recognizes the Peak Day with certainty.

IMPORTANT:
A constant discharge that is heavy, prolonged, irritating or offensive in odor, color and causes pain is abnormal and needs medical diagnosis. Abstinence is recommended until treatment has been completed so that the infection does not spread to the husband. The husband may also be treated, depending on the nature of the infection. If the woman is using a vaginal treatment the couple should abstain during treatment because it could disguise a fertile secretion.

Fertility is at its peak in the early twenties, after which it gradually declines. The decline in fertility is more marked from the late thirties onward. The fertility of the pre-menopausal woman is very much diminished.

As fertility declines, there is less mucus and so the PEAK DAY becomes less obvious. When this happens, the Early Day Rules are applied to every change from the B.I.P., including patches of mucus with a doubtful PEAK DAY, and any bleeding. Eventually bleeding and mucus will cease and the woman will be left with permanent infertility.

Following is an example of a pre-menopausal woman.

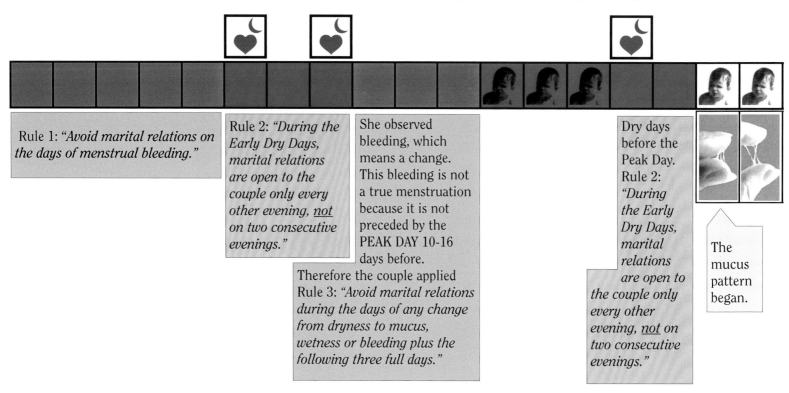

Rule 1: *"Avoid marital relations on the days of menstrual bleeding."*

Rule 2: *"During the Early Dry Days, marital relations are open to the couple only every other evening, not on two consecutive evenings."*

She observed bleeding, which means a change. This bleeding is not a true menstruation because it is not preceded by the PEAK DAY 10-16 days before.

Therefore the couple applied Rule 3: *"Avoid marital relations during the days of any change from dryness to mucus, wetness or bleeding plus the following three full days."*

Dry days before the Peak Day. Rule 2: *"During the Early Dry Days, marital relations are open to the couple only every other evening, not on two consecutive evenings."*

The mucus pattern began.

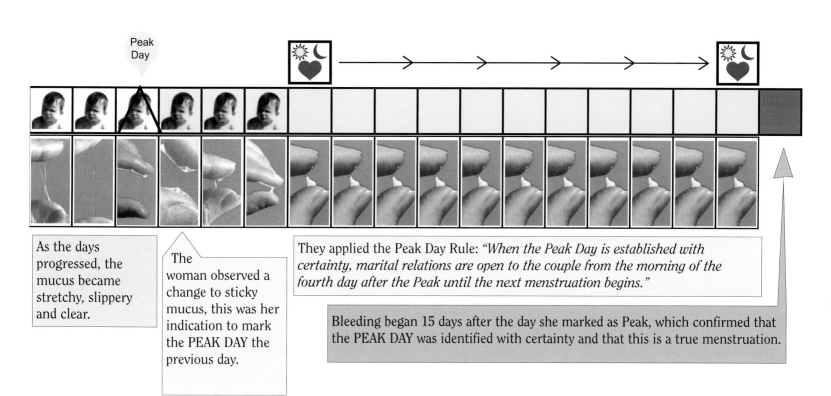

Peak Day

As the days progressed, the mucus became stretchy, slippery and clear.

The woman observed a change to sticky mucus, this was her indication to mark the PEAK DAY the previous day.

They applied the Peak Day Rule: *"When the Peak Day is established with certainty, marital relations are open to the couple from the morning of the fourth day after the Peak until the next menstruation begins."*

Bleeding began 15 days after the day she marked as Peak, which confirmed that the PEAK DAY was identified with certainty and that this is a true menstruation.

The Late Days of the cycle are called the Luteal Phase. This type of cycle with short luteal phase is present in special circumstances like pre-menopause and also during breastfeeding. It is important to note that to consider a woman under this circumstance, she must clearly identify her Peak Day. As mentioned before, to consider a bleeding as true menstruation there must be 10-16 days between the Peak Day and bleeding; these special circumstances during pre-menopause and breastfeeding are the exception.

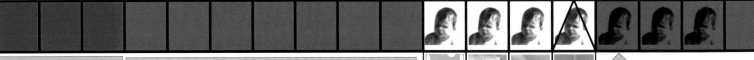

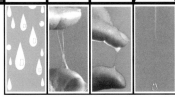

Rule 1: *"Avoid marital relations on the days of menstrual bleeding."*

She observed dry days. They applied Rule 2: *"During the Early Dry Days, marital relations are open to the couple only every other evening, <u>not</u> on two consecutive evenings."*

The mucus pattern began; the first day she didn't see anything but she felt wet. Then the mucus progressed to stretchy with a slippery sensation. They applied Rule 3: *"Avoid marital relations during the days of any change from dryness to mucus, wetness or bleeding plus the following three full days."*

She felt dry this day and marked the previous day as her Peak Day. They applied the Peak Day Rule: *"When the Peak Day is established with certainty, marital relations are open to the couple from the morning of the fourth day after the Peak until the next menstruation begins."*

This is an example of a short luteal phase cycle during pre-menopause. In this cycle she only had 8 days of luteal phase, this indicated that although she had probably ovulated, her cycle was infertile because the luteal phase was less than 10 days long. There was not enough build-up of nutrients in the endometrium to retain a pregnancy. Since she had identified the Peak Day, the couple could have marital relations any time, day or night until the next menstruation.

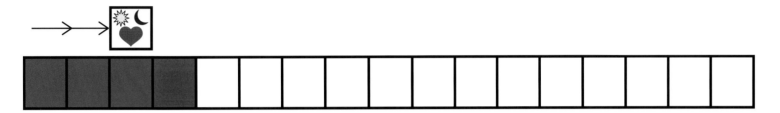

PRE-MENOPAUSE.

Pre-menopause may last 2-5 years prior to the cessation of menses; the woman's fertility is very much diminished. In order to avoid pregnancy, the woman must recognize infertility with a daily record for one month prior to applying the Ovulation Method. During pre-menopause, cycles could be normal; become irregular (extremely variable in length: short or long cycles); with intermittent bleeding; with patches of mucus that are increasingly less frequent and with a short luteal phase. A woman may ovulate infrequently or not at all, even though bleeding still occurs. Menses may be heavy and prolonged. A common infertile pattern for these women is dry, crusty, flaky mucus without the lubricative qualities of fertile-type mucus. She also can be dry, but remember that each woman has her own pattern. As fertility declines, there is less mucus and so the PEAK DAY becomes less obvious. When this happens, the Early Day Rules are applied to every change from the B.I.P. (including patches of mucus with a doubtful Peak Day and all bleeding). Eventually bleeding and mucus will cease and the woman will be left with a permanent B.I.P. of dryness indicating final infertility. In some women menstrual periods may stop without warning and not begin again.

Review

During Menstruation:

Avoid marital relations during the days of menstrual bleeding.

Reason 1: The bleeding could conceal the presence of mucus if the fertile phase begins early in the cycle.

Reason 2: There is medical support for abstinence during menstruation. There is evidence that women who engage in marital relations during menstruation increase their risk of endometriosis.

Early Dry Days:

Marital relations are open to the couple on alternate evenings of dry days immediately following menstruation. Dry days are defined as those when no mucus is seen and there is no feeling of wetness or lubrication.

Reason: Seminal fluid on the following morning after marital relations could conceal the presence of mucus. Marital relations are available to the couple on alternate evenings only since observations for any change from dryness should be made throughout the day.

The Fertile Phase:

At the first sign of change from dryness to the presence of mucus, or to a sensation of wetness or lubrication, the couple who wishes to postpone pregnancy must abstain from marital relations and genital contact until the PEAK DAY has been clearly identified, plus three full days following the PEAK DAY. Marital relations can be resumed on the morning of the fourth day after the PEAK DAY.

Reason: All mucus occurring prior to the PEAK DAY is considered fertile unless a Basic Infertile Pattern (B.I.P.) of mucus has been established.

See pages 84-87 and 98-99 for additional information about B.I.P.

The PEAK DAY:

The PEAK DAY is the last day that the mucus is stretchy, or a slippery wet sensation is felt at the vulva, even if mucus is not seen. This is not always the day when the quantity of the mucus is greatest, but the last day when any mucus with fertile characteristics is noticed, or a wet slippery sensation is felt during daily observations.

The PEAK DAY is identified the day after it occurs, when a change to sticky, non-elastic mucus or to dryness is observed. The correct identification of the PEAK DAY will be verified by menstruation occurring 10 to 16 days later.

Reason: Ovulation occurs on the PEAK DAY, or one to two days before or after the PEAK DAY. Sperm entry is possible into the uterus during the fertile phase and for three days after the PEAK DAY.

The Late Infertile Phase:

Count three days of dryness (or sticky, pasty mucus) after the PEAK DAY.
Relations are open to the couple any time, day or night from the morning of the 4th day until the next menstruation begins.

Reason: Ovulation usually takes place between PEAK DAY and the following day. Occasionally ovulation may take place two days after the PEAK DAY. The egg survives only between 12 and 24 hours, it then disintegrates and conception is impossible. Sperm can survive only when fertile cervical mucus is present in the woman's body. The cervix prevents sperm from entering the uterus by developing a thick mucus plug by the end of the third day after the PEAK DAY.

Additional guidelines for postponing pregnancy in special circumstances may be found on pages 96-103.

Note: Internal examination of the cervix to check for mucus or to check the position of the cervix *is unnecessary and is discouraged.* Observations are made by paying attention to any wet sensation felt. As the woman goes about her daily activities, she will feel the presence of the mucus similar to the way she feels her menstrual flow. The woman will also observe the mucus present when checking the bathroom tissue throughout the day. Vaginal douches should also be avoided, as they could destroy the natural protection in the vagina.

Natural vs Artificial

THE OVULATION METHOD OF NATURAL FAMILY PLANNING

1. The Ovulation Method is completely safe with no harmful side effects.

2. The Ovulation Method is simple to learn and to follow. It does not distort the marital act nor involve distasteful procedures. The spouses do nothing to their bodies but simply plan their marital relations according to the fertile and infertile days of the woman's cycle.

3. When used to postpone pregnancy, the Ovulation Method is more effective (98-99%) than any artificial method of birth control, but without the physical, psychological and spiritual side effects.

4. The Ovulation Method costs nothing more than the modest price of simple learning materials.

5. With the Ovulation Method, the woman is able to know herself, she learns to appreciate the normal processes of her own body.

6. Using the Ovulation Method enables the woman to accept and respect the gift of her fertility from the beginning to the end of her reproductive years.

7. The Ovulation Method fosters communication and mutual respect between husband and wife. The two cooperate in planning their family, taking into account the woman's normal functions of her reproductive cycle.

8. When the couple must postpone a pregnancy, the very abstinence that the Ovulation Method requires can help strengthen the marriage. The sacrifice involved is proof of the respect that the husband has for his wife. She in turn appreciates his willingness to sacrifice for her good and the good of the marriage, and the love for each other increases.

9. The love of the couple is renewed after a short period of abstinence with the Ovulation Method. Interest in the marital embrace is enhanced as well as generating a greater mutual love for each other.

10. The attitude of spouses who practice the Ovulation Method is: "Our fertility is a natural gift and a normal function of the human body." This helps to bring peace and greater intimacy to their relationship. When couples are required to abstain from marital relations for a few days each cycle (if they need to postpone pregnancy), they find other ways to express their love for each other. Communication increases, their love strengthens and they appreciate the gift of sexuality, experiencing a new honeymoon each month.

11. The Ovulation Method can be used to achieve as well as to postpone a pregnancy. It is immediately reversible when the couple changes their decision to achieve or postpone pregnancy.

12. The Ovulation Method is acceptable to people of all cultures, educational and social levels and religions. The spouses can use this natural method with a clear conscience. This method, when used generously and not for selfish or materialistic reasons, respects life and the privilege of transmitting life.

13. Studies confirm that the divorce rate is dramatically low among couples who practice the Ovulation Method of Natural Family Planning (see pages 122-133).

ARTIFICIAL METHODS OF BIRTH CONTROL

1. Every artificial birth control method involves medical risk. Therefore, it places a healthy woman at risk.

2. Artificial birth control involves ingesting dangerous drugs or using intrusive devices.

3. The more effective the artificial method, the more dangerous it is, e.g., the Pill, the Patch, Nuva-ring, Depo-Provera injection, Implants, Intrauterine Devices, etc.

4. Artificial birth control involves a continual expense.

5. Often artificial methods of birth control are used blindly without the woman knowing how they are affecting her body.

6. The use of artificial methods of birth control suppresses the normal, healthy functions of the human reproductive system.

7. The use of barrier methods such as condoms, diaphragms, spermicides, etc. do not always prevent conception when they are used in the 100 hours of fertility in the woman's cycle. It is critical for the couple to understand that while a woman can become pregnant for about 100 hours each cycle, venereal diseases can be transmitted at any time.

8. The use of artificial birth control often encourages spouses to never communicate with one another about something as important as bringing life into the world or postponing it. Most women are not even aware of when they are fertile or infertile.

9. Very often artificial birth control frees the man from any responsibility when it comes to planning a family. Most, if not all, of the burden of artificial birth control is placed on the woman.

10. Artificial birth control places a barrier between husband and wife and limits the most intense physical expression of human love. When the couple is never required to make the sacrifice of abstaining (as is the case while using artificial birth control), marital relations can lose their deeper meaning. It is easy for a husband and a wife to use each other instead of loving each other.

11. Prolonged use of artificial birth control sometimes results in infertility. For example, the Pill causes 150 chemical changes in the woman's body.

12. The level of discontent and the discontinuation rate of most artificial birth control methods is extremely high in many countries, especially in the Third World. Use of artificial birth control is unacceptable to many religious and cultural traditions because it involves a direct attack on the transmission of life. In addition, certain artificial birth control methods such as the Pill, the Patch, Nuva-ring, Depo-Provera injection, Implants, and Intrauterine Devices do not always prevent conception. Instead they can cause a very early abortion a few days later by preventing the newly conceived human person from implanting in the womb. Therefore they act as abortifacients.

13. The divorce rate among couples who use artificial birth control is much higher (See pages 122-133).

VIII.

Scientific Support of the
Ovulation Method

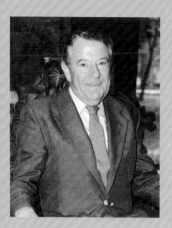

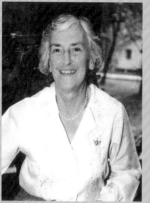

**John J. Billings
1918 - 2007
K.C.S.G., M.D.,
FRACP., FRCP. London**

Consulting Neurologist, St. Vincent's Hospital, Melbourne, Australia.

Member, St. Vincent's Bioethics Committee.

President of the World Organization of the Ovulation Method-Billings.

External examiner of uro-anatomy, University of Melbourne, Melbourne, Australia.

Chairman of the Medical Research Advisory Committee of the National Health and Medical Research Council of Australia.

Dean of the Undergraduate Medical School, St. Vincent's Hospital, Melbourne.

Evelyn L. Billings

**M.B., B.S., Melbourne
D.C.H., London**

Examiner in Histology and Embryology, Department of Anatomy, University of Melbourne, Australia.

Senior Consultant, Natural Family Planning Center, Department of Community Medicine, St. Vincent's Hospital, Melbourne, Australia.

Vice President of the World Organization of the Ovulation Method-Billings.

In the early 1950's, Dr. John Billings of Melbourne, Australia was asked to act as a medical advisor to couples who wished to use natural methods of family planning. The only natural methods then available were Rhythm and the Basal Body Temperature method. Both of these methods proved unreliable and unnecessarily limiting when the woman's cycles were long and irregular.

Dr. Billings went to the medical literature hoping to find a clue that would lead to the development of a better, more effective natural method. There he found references dating back to 1855 about a mucus secretion produced by the cervix of the uterus close to the time of ovulation. The physical and chemical properties of this secretion had been extensively studied but there were few references that this secretion was a familiar observation to healthy fertile women. He recognized the possible significance of the mucus as a marker of ovulation and wondered if this secretion could be used by women as a signal of fertility.

He then began to question a number of women about their observation of this secretion. They all confirmed that they had observed a mucus secretion during the menstrual cycle, but hadn't understood its significance. This was the clue he was looking for, the familiarity of healthy fertile women with the mucus secretion. It then became a matter of determining whether a typical mucus pattern existed during the cycle, and whether women could identify their fertile phase.

With the cooperation of hundreds of women, a standard mucus pattern quickly emerged. It became evident that the sensation produced by the mucus, as well as its appearance, could enable women to recognize the onset of fertility.

In 1962, Dr. Billings asked Dr. James Brown, an endocrinologist at the University of Melbourne, to conduct research correlating the accuracy of women's observations of the cervical mucus pattern with the ovarian hormonal patterns associated with ovulation. Dr. Brown agreed and thus there began a comprehensive program of combined clinical and laboratory research. Hundreds of women's cycles in all reproductive categories were tested. By 1964, the researchers were convinced that women's observations of their cervical mucus pattern identified their fertility as accurately as sophisticated laboratory tests.

The data from the research done by Brown and a number of his colleagues provided scientific verification of the new method, now called the Billings Ovulation Method or Ovulation Method. In 1964, Dr. Lyn Billings became involved in her husband's research. She began to train teachers and helped to refine and simplify the method.

In 1968 the author of this book Mercedes Arzu Wilson, learned the Ovulation Method from the Billings. At that time they also included the rhythm and temperature readings, now known as the Sympto-thermal Method. The research into the efficacy of the natural signs of cervical mucus during the fertile phase had just begun. Mrs. Wilson began teaching the Ovulation Method in Guatemala to the poor and illiterate people, trying for the first time to use it only with the signs of cervical mucus with a chart and stamps of different colors. As the successful use of the chart and stamps increased, Mrs. Wilson invited doctors Billings to Guatemala, other countries of Central America and Mexico. When they studied the evidence of the effectiveness of the simple charting system, they decided to incorporate it for their instructors around the world, and to eliminate the rhythm and temperature readings. The simplification of the Ovulation Method helped its rapid expansion throughout the world.

The Ovulation Method can be used both to achieve and postpone pregnancy. When used to achieve pregnancy, a couple of normal fertility will usually conceive within three cycles. When used to postpone pregnancy, the Ovulation Method has an effectiveness rate of 98-99%.

Dr. John Billings died in 2007, having left a historic legacy in the field of N.F.P.

Effectiveness Studies of the Ovulation Method

Study	Country	Year	Couples	Cycles Duration	* Method Related Pregnancies	References
Billings, J	Australia	1972	165	1,560	0.00%	*J. Irish Med*. Assoc. 70 (Apr. 1977):6.
Weissman, SR. M	Tonga	1972	282	2,503	0.50%	*Lancet*, 2 (1972): 813-16.
Billings, L. Premenopause	Australia	1972	98	3-4 years	0.00%	"The Billings Method" - Edited by Anne O'Donovan, Pty, Ltd., Australia.
St. Cloud	U.S.A	1974	260	1,823	0.60%	Human Life Foundation Newsletter, March, 1974.
Ball, M.	Australia	1976	124	1,635	2.90%	Europe, *J. Ob. Gyn & Rep. Biol*. 6 (1976): 2, 63-66.
Kyu San Cho	Korea	1976	Urban: 465 Rural: 918	11,064	Urban: 1.61% Rural: 1.96%	W.H.O. Meeting, Geneva February, 1976.
Happy Family Movement	Korea	1977-78	3,806	24,414	1.40%	Annual Report, H.F.M., Korea, 1977-78, p. 1-4.
World Health Organization	Philippines, India, El Salvador, New Zealand, Ireland	1977-78	725	7,514	2.80%	*Fert. Ster*., Vol. 36, Pg. 591, 1981.
Mascarenhas	India	1978	3,530	39,967	0.06%	Mascarenhas M.M., "The use-effectiveness of the Ovulation Method in India", 9:209, 1979.
Dolack, L.	U.S.A.	1978	329	3,354	1.10%	Hosp. Program (Aug. 1978), p. 64 FF.
Tamil Nadu F.L. Center, Bernard, C	India	1978-79	3,275	39,300	0.00%	Annual Reports 1978-1985.
Cilacap Rural	Indonesia	1978-82	978	14,541	0.27%	Pusat Metode Ovulasi, Jl. Jen. A. Yani 23, Cilacap.
Klaus, H. et.al.	U.S.A.	1979	1,090	12,282	1.17%	*Contraception*, 19 (June 1979): 6.
Klaus, H.	U.S.A.	1981	72	808	0.00%	Presented 9th Annual Conference on Psychosomatic Ob. Gyn. 1981
A. Dedé	Italy (Lombardia)	1985	720	2,975	0.00%	Medicina e Morale, Jan, 1985.
Xu, J.X. Zhang D.W.	People's Rep. of China	1988-90	688	11,075	1.18%	Presented at 16th International Congress for the Family, Brighton, England, 1990.
Ryder, R.E.J.	India (Calcutta)	1993	19,843	6,467	0.40%	*British Medical Journal*, Sept. 18, 1993, 307:723-6.
Wilson, M.	Guatemala	1997-99	937	10,872	0.65%	Presented at The Knights of Malta Medical Assoc., Jan. 2002.
Wilson, M.	Guatemala	2007-10	506	3,341	0.00%	Presented at International Institute of Restorative Reproductive Medicine, Jul. 2010.

* Method-related pregnancies are those which occur despite correct application of the rules for pregnancy avoidance. This chart reports method-related pregnancies only, for purposes of this presentation. The Ovulation Method will provide this high effectiveness only when couples fully abstain from sexual relations during the fertile phase. Couples who use barrier methods or have genital contact during the time of fertility risk a high pregnancy rate.

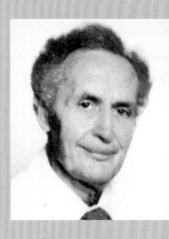

James B. Brown
1919 - 2009

Degrees and Fellowships

M.Sc. (1st Class Honours),
New Zealand University, 1940.

Ph.D., University of Edinburgh, 1952.
D.Sc., University of Edinburgh, 1970.

Fellow of the Royal Australian College of Obstetricians
and Gynecologists.

Professor Emeritus and Associate,
Department of Obstetrics and Gynecology,
Royal Women's Hospital, University of Melbourne.

The late Dr. Brown worked since 1947 on the application of hormone assays in the identification of the phases of fertility and infertility during the menstrual cycle in Auckland, New Zealand; in Edinburgh, Scotland (1949-1962) and in Melbourne, Australia (1962-2009). In Edinburgh he was involved in the development of the first accurate hormone assays for estrogens, pregnanediol and total gonadotrophins in urine, and later, in Melbourne, refined the assays for estrogens and pregnanediol for rapid and mass application. During the 1960s, Dr. Brown used these assays in helping Drs. John and Lyn Billings develop and validate the Ovulation Method.

He was involved in the international application of hormone assays in cancer research and, with his colleagues at Harvard University, he was awarded the 1986 Antoine Lecassagne prize by *La Ligue Nationale Francaise contre le Cancer*. He was also involved with Georgetown University, U.S.A.I.D. and Family Health International, in a large multinational study of returning fertility in breastfeeding women.

SCIENTIFIC VERIFICATION OF THE OVULATION METHOD

Much of the early key research into the Ovulation Method was carried out by Dr. James Brown. In 1962, Dr. Billings asked Dr. Brown to conduct hormonal studies to correlate the accuracy of women's observations of the cervical mucus patterns associated with ovulation. Dr. Brown agreed and began a comprehensive program of clinical and laboratory research. Hundreds of women's cycles in all reproductive categories were tested.

Dr. Brown's research showed that the development of the mucus symptom coordinated with the estrogen levels in the follicular phase of the cycle much better than any other symptom accompanying ovulation; it also helped establish the relationship between estrogen and progesterone, the cervical mucus changes and ovulation.

While Dr. Brown worked on estrogen and progesterone, his colleague, Dr. Henry Burger, an endocrinologist at Monash University, Melbourne, worked on the other hormones which regulate the menstrual cycle: *Follicle Stimulating Hormone* (FSH) which stimulates the development of the follicle containing the ovum; and *Luteinizing Hormone* (LH) which triggers ovulation.

Using blood samples provided by the Ovulation Method users, Professor Burger was able to chart the changes in LH and FSH during the cycles of normally fertile women. He was able to show the relationship of the peak mucus symptom and the LH peak. Professors Brown and Burger, working with Dr. Kevin Catt[1], showed that the release of LH followed the mid-cycle estrogen peak by a mean 16 hours (range 0-2 days).

The work of Drs. Billings, Brown and Burger[2] relating hormone changes to the mucus symptom was first published in a British medical journal, the *Lancet*, in 1972. This study showed that the time of ovulation could be identified by women themselves when charting their mucus symptom without recourse to either basal body temperature measurement or more specialized tests. The study established the relationship between the surge of LH, ovulation, and the observation of the peak mucus symptom.

Further studies[3] of these relationships have been conducted under the direction of the World Health Organization's expanded program of research, development, and research training in human reproduction. The available evidence indicates that:

– The estradiol spurt resulting in fertile-type mucus that warns of possible fertility, starts on average six days before ovulation.

– The estradiol peak occurs about thirty-seven hours before ovulation.

– The LH level begins to rise about thirty to forty hours before ovulation, reaching a peak about seventeen hours before the ovum is released.

– The peak mucus symptom, as judged by women themselves, occurs on average 0.6 day (fourteen hours) before ovulation. In about 85 percent of women the Peak occurs within a day of ovulation and in about 95 percent within two days[4].

– 93% of the subjects in one WHO study were able to identify an interpretable ovulatory mucus pattern in the first teaching cycle[5].

NOTES

1. "Relationship between plasma luteinizing hormone and urinary estrogen excretion during the menstrual cycle," H.G. Burger, K.J. Catt and J.B. Brown, *Journal of clin. Endocrin. and Metab.* 28:1508-1512, 1968.

2. "Symptoms and hormonal changes accompanying ovulation," E.L. Billings, J.J. Billings, J.B. Brown and H.G. Burger, *Lancet* 1:282-284, 1972.

3. "Cervical mucus, the biological marker of fertility and infertility," J.J. Billings, *International Journal of Fertility* 26:182-195, 1981.

4. World Health Organization Colloquium, "The Cervical Mucus in Human Reproduction," Geneva, 1972.

5. World Health Organization, "A prospective Multicenter Trial of the Ovulation Method of Natural Family Planning. II. The Effectiveness Phase," *Fertility and Sterility*, 36, 591, 1981.

The results of 850,000 hormone assays were obtained by Dr. Brown in collaboration with colleagues and reported in more than 220 publications in referred journals and chapters of books. This is equivalent to one publication every two months for nearly 40 years! The 850,000 assays were mainly daily urinary estrogen and pregnanediol measurements throughout at least 12,000 menstrual cycles[6].

Women who may have difficult mucus symptoms, such as those breastfeeding, discontinuing the Pill or approaching menopause, will find the kit most helpful in supplying absolute markers of fertility and infertility.

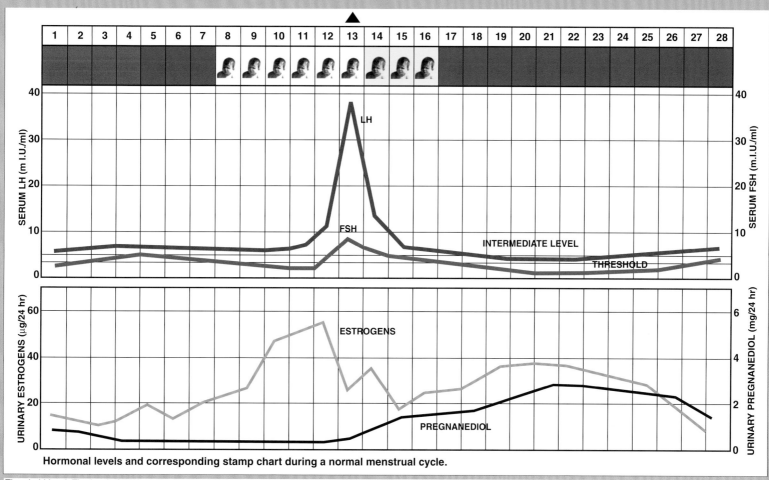

Hormonal levels and corresponding stamp chart during a normal menstrual cycle.

Threshold level: The level of FSH required by the follicles to be stimulated into active growth. While they grow, they produce estradiol.
Intermediate Level: The level of LH that must be reached to boost one of the growing follicles into completing the whole process of ovulation. If this level is exceeded, then multiple ovulations are likely to occur. It is only 20% above the threshold level.

The "Continuum"

According to Dr. Brown, many variants of the 28 day ovulatory cycle may occur:[7]

- Ovulatory cycles as short as 19 days are due to very early rising of FSH.

- Long ovulatory cycles are due to delayed FSH production.

- Anovulation, when follicle develops but does not progress to ovulation. There is production of estrogen which later decreases. Depending on the amount of estrogen produced and the sensitivity of the endometrium, the decrease in estrogen levels may or may not produce bleeding (withdrawal bleeding). There may be fertile days that do not progress to PEAK DAY because there was no ovulation.

- Anovulation, when many follicles remain stimulated and produce constant raised levels of estrogen. If these raised levels persist, the endometrium may break down producing bleeding (breakthrough bleeding). These women may experience a B.I.P. of constant discharge.

- Luteinized Unruptured Follicle (LUF). The follicle is boosted towards ovulation, but there is no ovulation because there is very little amount of LH, not sufficient to cause rupture (ovulation). There is only a small quantity of progesterone; the woman has fertile secretion but no PEAK DAY.

- Ovulation occurs but cycle is infertile. In this variant, LH surge is sufficient to cause ovulation but not enough to support a pregnancy:
a) Progesterone rise does not reach the levels to support a pregnancy; this is called "Deficient Luteal phase". It may be associated with difficulty in recognizing the Peak Day.
b) Progesterone levels reach normal post-ovulatory values but fall prematurely so that bleeding occurs 10 days or less after ovulation; this is called "Short Luteal Phase". It is recognized by a shortened interval between the PEAK DAY and menstruation.

Both cycles are ovulatory but infertile.

NOTES

6. Billings, E.L., Billings, J.J., Brown, J.B., and Burguer, H.G., Symptoms and Hormonal Changes Accompanying Ovulation, Lancet 1:282-284, 1972.

7. Brown, J.B., Ovarian Activity and Fertility and the Billings Ovulation Method, 2005. WOOMB.

8. Brown J.B., Harrison P., Smith M.A., Burger H.G., "Correlations between the mucus symptoms and the hormonal markers of fertility throughout reproductive life", Monograph, Advocate Press, Melbourne, 1981.

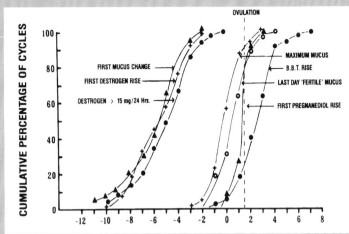

This graph was used by Dr. Billings in a study published in 1981 in the *International Journal of Fertility*[3]. It illustrates the correlation between changes in mucus, basal body temperature, and pregnanediol in 43 cycles, further confirms that cervical mucus, as charted by women themselves, accurately reflects what is taking place in the ovary. Day of cycle relative to estrogen peak = day 0. The vertical broken line shows the approximate time of ovulation.[8]

Urinary estrogen and pregnanediol values, mucus symptoms, and basal temperature during three cycles in a normal subject.

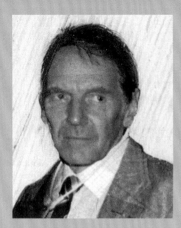

Erik Odeblad, M.D., Ph.D.

Professor and Chairman of the
Department of Medical Biophysics,
University of Umeå, Sweden, and
former research fellow of the Swedish
Medical Research Council, Department of
Obstetrics and Gynecology, Karolinska
Institute, Sabbatsberg Hospital, Stockholm,
Sweden.

Cervical mucus is a complex secretion produced constantly by the mucus secreting epithelial cells of the endocervix. There are approximately 400 mucus-secreting glandular-like units (crypts) in the cervical canal which produce mucus at the rate of 20 to 60 mg per day in normal women of reproductive age. During midcycle, the amount increases tenfold and may reach up to 700 mg per day.

The most important constituent of cervical mucus is a hydrogel, rich in carbohydrates and consisting of glycoproteins of the mucin type (A glycoprotein is one of a group of protein-carbohydrate compounds among which are the mucins; a mucin is a proteinaceous material which when combined with water forms mucus). Most of the physical properties of cervical mucus are due to mucins.

Cyclic alterations in the consistency of cervical mucus influence sperm penetrability, nutrition, and survival. Optimal changes of cervical mucus properties, such as greatest increase in quantity, spinnbarkeit, ferning and pH, and decrease in viscosity and cell content, occur immediately prior to ovulation, and are reversed after ovulation.[1]

Pre-ovulatory mucus is most receptive to sperm penetration.

The secretion of cervical mucus is regulated by the ovarian hormones. The components of the cervical mucus change markedly during the cycle, reflecting the preponderance of estrogens or progesterone. The secretion of different types of mucus and, accordingly, their biophysical properties (i.e., spinnbarkeit, crystallization, and consistency) are largely determined by these hormonal factors.

The structure and function of the mucus and its relation to fertility and infertility have been most thoroughly investigated by Dr. Erik Odeblad and his colleagues at the University of Umeå in Sweden. The following are some of their findings:

1. The key to nearly all the present research was the discovery, first published in 1976, that there are three types of cervical mucus, G, L and S.

G mucus seals the cervical canal during the infertile days of the cycle. It is present in one variety immediately after menstruation, in another during the post-ovulatory phase of the cycle, and probably in a third during pregnancy.

The post-menstrual G mucus is supplanted by L mucus when the circulating estrogens rise. The L mucus, the first mucus symptom of the cycle is a soft, mucinous secretion which turns into a slippery, watery secretion a few days before ovulation when S mucus is produced. The S mucus, the sperm receptive mucus, provides low viscosity channels for the sperm by which they gain access into the cervix and uterine cavity. A certain balance between the S and L secretion seems to be necessary for optimum fertility. Shortly after ovulation, both L and S mucus disappear and the post-ovulatory G mucus appears.

2. The ovulatory mucus is a mosaic made up of mucus strings and mucus loaves. The strings contain the fluid gel, S mucus, and the loaves the more viscid gel, L mucus. The S mucus is very thin and flows rapidly between the loaves of L mucus. The strings are about 100 μm (microns) in diameter and 2-3 cm long. The loaves are ellipsoid and 0.3 x 1 x 3 mm in size. Near the external os, there are some units of still more viscid G mucus.

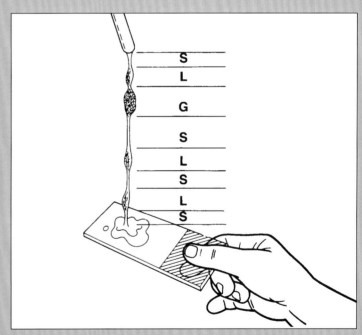

When performing the spinnbarkeit test, one can see that the mucus thread is uneven due to the presence of different types of cervical secretions. The S and L types are transparent, the G type is opalescent. The thin parts of the thread denote the S mucus.

The S secretion composes approximately 30 percent of midcycle mucus and the L secretion 70 percent, although there is a day-to-day percentage variation due to the continuous secretion and outflow of the mucus.

3. The ellipsoid units of L mucus provide the mechanical framework for the fluid S mucus and act as a trapping mechanism for sperm which are presumably not suitable for conception.

4. S and L mucus are produced by different secreting areas of the endocervix. The upper part of the cervix tends to secrete most of the S mucus. The peak symptom of the mucus discharge coincides sometimes, but not always, with the maximum of the slippery S mucus secretion.

5. The time around ovulation when the S mucus is produced seems to be age dependent. In young women the S mucus is normally present for a longer time. At the age of about 20 years, the average time for S mucus secretion is about 4-5 days, while at 35 years, the average time is only about 1-2 days. A statistically significant correlation up to the age of about 35 years has been found. Also the spinnbarkeit changes with age in a similar but more complicated way.

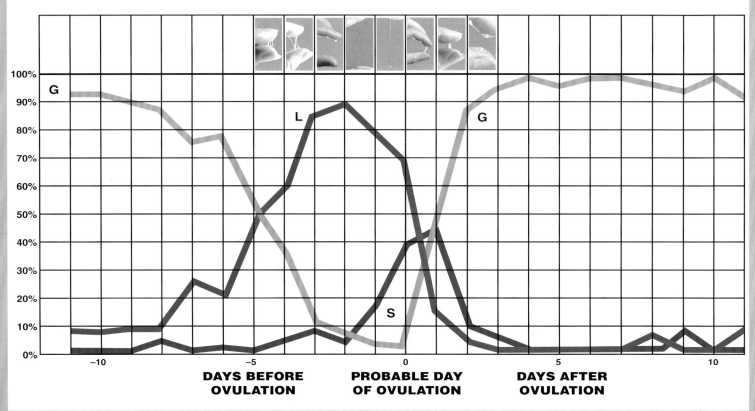

The cyclic variation of percentage of G, L, and S mucus based on 1,124 cervical samples. Immediately after menstruation the G type dominates. When the estrogen stimulus on the cervical mucosa increases, the mucosa responds with increased L secretion. The S mucus does not increase until 1-2 days before ovulation and is actually high also the day after ovulation when it then decreases suddenly. The L mucus decreases about one day before the S mucus. During the corpus luteum phase, the G mucus dominates. The day after ovulation, the G mucus is secreted from crypts in the lowest part of the cervix and the external os. This aids to close the cervical canal at its lower end. Above this "closed door" there is a very loose or liquid mucus "plug" consisting mainly of S mucus and containing the sperm released from the crypts which have been colonized during the first phase of sperm advance. The whole upper part of the cervical canal now acts as a big sperm reservoir, capable of continuously exposing the ovum to sperm.[2]

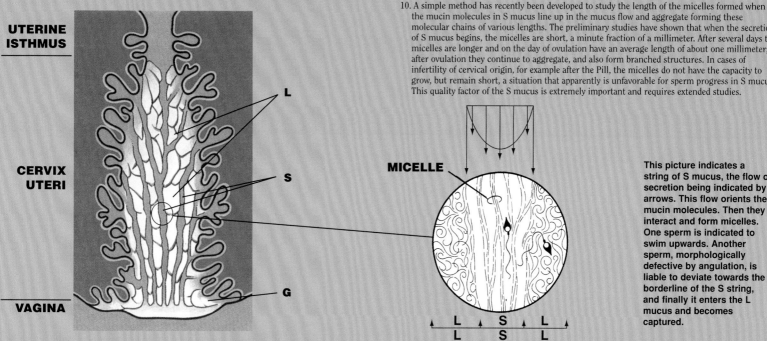

UTERINE ISTHMUS

CERVIX UTERI

L

S

G

VAGINA

MICELLE

L S L
L S L

10. A simple method has recently been developed to study the length of the micelles formed when the mucin molecules in S mucus line up in the mucus flow and aggregate forming these molecular chains of various lengths. The preliminary studies have shown that when the secretion of S mucus begins, the micelles are short, a minute fraction of a millimeter. After several days the micelles are longer and on the day of ovulation have an average length of about one millimeter; after ovulation they continue to aggregate, and also form branched structures. In cases of infertility of cervical origin, for example after the Pill, the micelles do not have the capacity to grow, but remain short, a situation that apparently is unfavorable for sperm progress in S mucus. This quality factor of the S mucus is extremely important and requires extended studies.

This picture indicates a string of S mucus, the flow of secretion being indicated by arrows. This flow orients the mucin molecules. Then they interact and form micelles. One sperm is indicated to swim upwards. Another sperm, morphologically defective by angulation, is liable to deviate towards the borderline of the S string, and finally it enters the L mucus and becomes captured.

6. Studies on the dose-response curve for the L and S mucus on estrogenic stimulation indicate that the L mucus requires only low doses of estrogen in circulating blood, while the S mucus requires higher levels. This finding easily explains why L mucus occurs before the S mucus in the normal cycle. But it is still not understood why the S mucus can be produced when the estrogen levels decrease after the estrogen peak. This is presently being studied in detail.[3]

7. The flow of S mucus orients the mucin molecules, which then tend to form long thin aggregates, called micelles, separated by a waterlike medium, which permit very rapid sperm advance.

8. The anatomy of the mucus mosaic is such that some sperm swim to the uterine cavity, but most move to the S secreting crypts in which they seem to hibernate and form a sperm reservoir with a half-time of about 15 hours.

9. The advance of high-quality sperm seems to be a highly ordered process, in formal agreement with mathematical group theory. This indicates that some kind of intercommunication between the sperm cells exists, phonons being the carriers of intercellular messages.

11. Post-IUD inflammatory conditions and other similar sequelae of sexually transmitted diseases, many of which have been promoted by the use of the Pill, are also being studied. It seems that inflammatory conditions may influence the capacity of the cervix to produce mucus of good quality. In depth studies in this particular field have not yet been conducted.

NOTES

1. Odeblad, Erik, The Biophysical Properties of the Cervical-Vaginal Secretions, Int Rev Nat Fam Pla, 7:1-56, 1983

2. Billings, E.L., and J.J., Catarinich, M., Billings Atlas of the Ovulation Method, p.85-94, 1989

3. Odeblad, Erik, Some Notes on the Cervical Crypts, Bulletin of the Ovulation Method Research and Reference Centre of Australia, Vol 24 No 2, p. 312, June 1997.

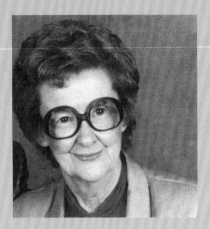

Ruth S. Taylor, M.D.
1924-2011

Medical Director, Natural Family
Planning, St. Francis Hospital,
Wichita, Kansas.

Head, Cytogenetics Section,
St. Francis Hospital, Wichita, Kansas.

Cytopathologist,
St. Francis Hospital,
Wichita, Kansas.

Medical Director and Program Director,
St. Francis Hospital School of
Cytotechnology, Wichita, Kansas.

COMPOSITE OF THE MENSTRUAL CYCLE

The composite of the various processes which make up a woman's menstrual cycle is reminiscent of the musical score for a symphony orchestra. Recall, if you will, that each line of an orchestra's score represents the part for each instrument to follow and, as each instrument performs its designated role, a harmonious composition will be rendered. So, too, with the menstrual cycle.

OVARIAN CYCLE

Ovulation is the paramount event in the menstrual cycle and is a function of the ovary. All of the menstrual processes focus on this fantastic event, which indicates the optimum time for pregnancy. Contrary to some textbooks which claim that ovulation occurs on the 14th day of the cycle, ovulation actually takes place approximately 14 days before the subsequent menstrual flow, regardless of the length of the cycle.

PITUITARY AND OVARIAN HORMONES

Ovulation is orchestrated by the hypothalamus of the brain through the pituitary hormones, follicle stimulating hormone [FSH] and luteinizing hormone [LH], and the ovarian hormones, estrogen and progesterone. These four hormones interplay in a series of crescendos and decrescendos to insure the proper stimulation for the ripened ovum to wander from its family home and be captured by the Fallopian tube where it will lie in wait for its conqueror. The interaction of these hormones assures that the ovulatory event will not repeat itself in the same cycle. This is accomplished through feedback mechanisms causing the rising ovarian estrogens to peak and abruptly precipitate and allow LH to spike like a crashing cymbal triggering the eruption of the ovum from the follicle 16 hours later.

BASAL BODY TEMPERATURE (BBT)

Due to the performance of progesterone, which rises rapidly in the corpus luteum following ovulation, the basal body temperature (BBT) also becomes elevated after ovulation, indicating a slightly increased metabolism and providing a warmer environment for the developing new life should pregnancy occur.

VAGINAL CELLS KARYOPYKNOTIC INDEX (KPI)

Even the vaginal lining performs in this cyclic menstrual review, becoming thick, lush, and most protective near ovulation in response to estrogens, which alone can mature the vaginal epithelial cells. By evaluating the ratio of mature to immature cell forms microscopically in vaginal smears this maturation can be indicated by what is known as the Karyopyknotic Index (KPI). KPI peak reflects the estrogen peak near ovulation.

LEUKOCYTES (WHITE CELLS)

Leukocytes or white cells are common inhabitants of the cervical-vaginal tract as a part of the body's defense mechanism by phagocytizing predators. Sperm are one of those predators they readily destroy. Interestingly, leukocytes essentially disappear in the cervical mucus and the vagina near ovulation (another function of the mature vaginal epithelium). Hence, the chance of more sperm reaching their goal in the Fallopian tube is made less difficult during this critical time.

CERVICAL MUCUS

Without a doubt, the greatest assistance given sperm during their long arduous and amorous journey, is provided by the cervical mucus, whose role is to perform like a biological valve, facilitating passage, providing nourishment, storage and release of selected sperm when the objective, the ovum, is ready and waiting to be pursued. At other times during the menstrual cycle, the mucus, changed in response to progesterone secretion or before estrogen stimulation, effectively blocks the passage of sperm from entering the cervix. Women using the Ovulation Method can accurately identify their fertile phase. The peak mucus symptom defined by the Ovulation Method rules is not surpassed by any of the other ovulatory indicators mentioned above: pituitary or ovarian hormones, BBT or KPI.

SUMMARY

The spectacular and complex symphonic poem which represents the woman's fertility, composed of components of the menstrual cycle, will function normally in the majority of women, with proper care. Conversely, fertility can be harmed by many things and, in today's society, the opposite is too often the case, i.e. many women's menstrual functions have been damaged, frequently permanently, by sexually transmitted diseases, drugs, devices and surgical sterilizing procedures. Appreciation of the precious gift of fertility, i.e. men and women's ability to give life to another human person of equal value to themselves, can best be assured by cooperation with the natural processes of their reproductive physiology. Natural Family Planning offers this opportunity.

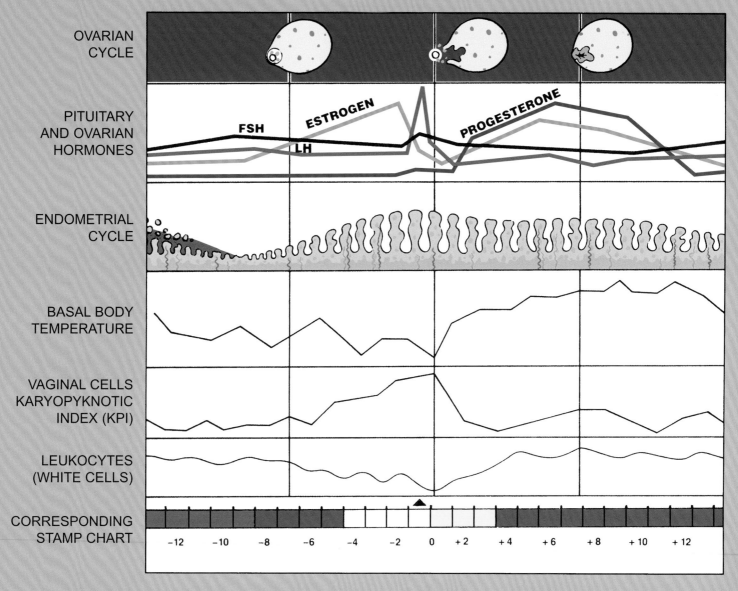

OVARIAN CYCLE

PITUITARY AND OVARIAN HORMONES

FSH

ESTROGEN

LH

PROGESTERONE

ENDOMETRIAL CYCLE

BASAL BODY TEMPERATURE

VAGINAL CELLS KARYOPYKNOTIC INDEX (KPI)

LEUKOCYTES (WHITE CELLS)

CORRESPONDING STAMP CHART

-12   -10   -8   -6   -4   -2   0   +2   +4   +6   +8   +10   +12

IX.

Natural vs. Artificial Birth Control

SUMMARY OF THE STUDY ON THE PRACTICE OF NATURAL FAMILY PLANNING VERSUS THE USE OF ARTIFICIAL BIRTH CONTROL: FAMILY, SEXUAL AND MORAL ISSUES

By Mercedes Arzú Wilson

Introduction

For many years, research has pointed to substantial differences between couples who practice Natural Family Planning (NFP) and couples who use artificial birth control. Using data collected from a sample of women in the United States of America who practice Natural Family Planning and comparing them to well-known national surveys, this study examined the effects of Natural Family Planning and artificial birth control on several dimensions of marital and family life. The study found that NFP women have lower rates of abortion and a dramatic low divorce rate (0.2%), than women in the national samples who use artificial birth control. The NFP women are more likely to be married and are more likely to recommend premarital chastity to young women. It was also interesting to note that couples who practice NFP had more marital relations, had more children and enjoyed greater happiness in their life than those using artificial birth control. The study also finds a high level of success in family life among NFP women, as well as a strong religious faith. Results support the hypothesis that Natural Family Planning is associated with positive spousal relationships and family stability. Interpretations of new data are discussed.

Natural Family Planning

It is essential to understand what is meant by Natural Family Planning in order to realize why it produces so many benefits to the marriage. In general, Natural Family Planning (NFP) is defined as methods for achieving or postponing pregnancy that are based on observations of naturally occurring signs in the woman's body that inform her of the fertile and infertile phases of her cycle. Authentic Natural Family Planning never interferes with the transmission of life; its sincere openness to the Will of God and respect for life is its most vital virtue. Various natural methods are being taught throughout the world that respect the Natural Law and are accepted by most cultures and religions. The Ovulation Method (OM) of Natural Family Planning is at present the most widely used method because it is the easiest to learn and simplest to follow.

The NFP survey participants in the following study were generally practicing the Ovulation Method. This method is neither the old "Rhythm" method nor the "Temperature" or Sympto-Thermal Method. It is based on the simple recognition of natural signs of fertility that appear for a few days during a woman's fertile cycle (see Figure 1). It is important to recognize that a woman is only fertile for approximately 100 hours per cycle during her reproductive years, whereas a man is potentially fertile every day from puberty onward. The advantages of the OM that influence the practice of Natural Family Planning within the marriage are not only spiritual, such as increased church attendance and frequency of prayer, but also psychological and physical.

The Ovulation Method is simple to learn and safe to practice and does not depend on regularity of cycles for its effectiveness. It has no physical side effects, and it does not interfere with the conjugal act nor does it involve distasteful procedures. When practiced to postpone pregnancy, it is 98-99% effective, even among the poorest of the poor in developing countries,[1] or among couples of no religious persuasion, as in China[2] (*see Figure 2*). When asked how satisfied they were with communication with their spouse, 88% of the NFP women responded positively. The high level of communication between spouses is without a doubt the fundamental ingredient that contributes to the success of any marriage. As this sharing and bonding develops, both husband and wife embrace mutual responsibility in deciding to postpone or bring new life into the world each cycle. It is not surprising, therefore, that the divorce rate among couples who practice NFP is extremely low. Women discover signs of fertility never fully understood or taught before. The OM has also proven extremely helpful in assisting seemingly infertile couples to conceive a baby. It fosters communication and mutual respect between the spouses as they accept responsibility in their decision to achieve or postpone pregnancy. It seems to bring peace and greater intimacy to the marriage. When practiced generously and not for selfish or materialistic reasons, the spouses respect life and the privilege given to them of transmitting life.

Figure 1 depicts the simplicity of the OM by teaching women to recognize the natural signs of her fertility comparing it to the fertility and infertility of the land.

Artificial Birth Control

In contrast, couples who use artificial methods of birth control seem to experience disturbing spiritual and psychological as well as physical risks to their body and soul. The normal functions of the woman's body are disrupted by the ingestion of dangerous chemicals or the use of mechanical devices (see pages 136-176 for health implications of artificial birth control methods). Often the woman is not informed of the internal effects on her body, nor of the abortifacient effect of most artificial methods of birth control (the Pill, *Norplant*,* the Patch, *Nuva Ring*, *Depo-Provera* injections, Intrauterine Devices), as they interfere with the normal growth and development of the endometrial lining,

Figure 1

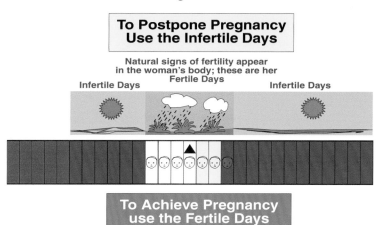

Figure 2

Effectiveness Rates of NFP in the United States, Guatemala, and the People's Republic of China

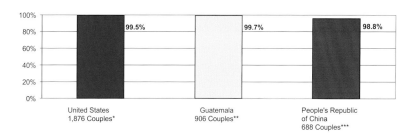

*Hilgers, Thomas W., M.D. and Stanford, Joseph B., M.D., M.S.P.H., "Creighton Model NaProEducation Technology for Avoiding Pregnancy - Use Effectiveness", June 1998, Vol 43, Number 6.

**Familia de las Americas, Presentation given at Knights of Malta, New York, 2001.

***Dr. Zhang D.W. and J.X. Xu "The Effectiveness of the Ovulation Method", Reproduction and Contraception, 1993 vol. 13, No 3 p. 194-200.

turning it hostile to the implantation of a new human life already conceived a few days earlier.

* *Norplant* is no longer available in the U.S., yet it is still in use in poor countries.[3]

Methodology of Data Collection

The data used to examine the NFP study came from a survey conducted during the summer and fall of 2000 by Family of the Americas Foundation (FAF), an international, educational non-profit organization that promotes NFP. Sampling for the NFP study was not random, although the investigator did attempt to generate a representative sample of women in the U.S. who practice NFP. Participants were drawn from 31 states, making the NFP sample national in scope.

Sample Characteristics

The comparison results in different parts of this study are from three distinct sources: 1) a survey conducted by Family of the Americas Foundation, directed by an independent evaluator. This is the first-ever survey of its kind to examine the impact of Natural Family Planning on a wide variety of family, marital, sexual and moral issues; 2) the National Survey of Family Growth (NSFG) which was carried out by the U.S. Government's National Center for Health Statistics; and 3) the General Social Survey (GSS) conducted by the National Opinion Research Center.

The NFP survey asked questions of 505 couples 21 to 66 years of age; the National Survey of Family Growth (NSFG) queried 10,847 women 15 to 44 years; the General Social Survey (GSS) questioned 19,786 women 18 years of age and older; and the sub-group Ever Married Catholic (EMC) pertains only to GSS respondents who are Catholic, and who have been married at some time in their lives (including those who are currently married). Another sub-group from the NSFG survey was also analyzed that compared Catholics from the NFP survey and Catholics from the NSFG survey who ranged in age from 21 to 44. These sub-groups, both Catholics within the same age range, gave us an especially useful, more controlled comparison.

HOW ABORTION, DIVORCE, AND PROMISCUITY ARE LINKED TO THE USE OF ARTIFICIAL BIRTH CONTROL

The statistical connections are becoming clear. Abortion, divorce, and multiple sexual partners are all statistically associated with the use of artificial birth control. Abstinence before marriage and chastity within, is not only the message taught with Natural Family Planning, it is the essential message that should be taught to young men and women before they become entrenched in the dominant artificial birth control mentality that is so harmful to the Sacrament of Matrimony and the welfare of the family.

In our thirty-six years of experience, seldom have we counseled couples that have not been wounded by the experience of using artificial birth control. They are surprised and often angry at not having been privy to such vital and simple knowledge as NFP earlier in their lives. Artificial birth control has affected the physical and spiritual health of many couples who end up aborting their child and divorcing their spouse. This supports the conclusion that the consequences of violating the Natural Law has been to the detriment of their matrimonial vows.

Even though 91% of the couples in our survey were Catholic, most of them (65%) had violated Church teaching on artificial birth control, 32% had numerous sexual partners since age 18 and 5% of the women had induced abortions. Nevertheless, as we study their replies in the survey, a change of heart appears to have taken place in their married life and seems to correlate with the practice of Natural Family Planning.

Divorce Rates in the General Population

Even though our NFP survey is not a random sample, but is national in scope, the NSFG and GSS surveys were random. The following graph illustrates the current marital status of all three studies as well as that of the sub-sample of the GSS Ever Married Catholics. However, a definitive comparison cannot be made because of the age difference among the NFP (21 to 66), the NSFG (15 to 44), the GSS and the GSS Ever Married Catholic (18 and older), survey groups. Nevertheless, the adjusted comparisons reported later in this summary provide more precise results.

Figure 3: NFP, NSFG, GSS and GSS Ever Married Catholics Data

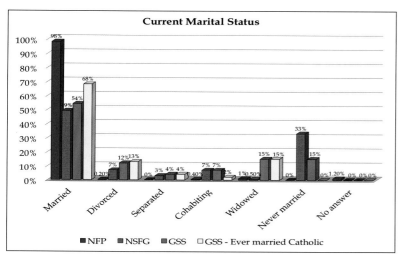

At the time of the surveys, 98% of NFP, 49% of the NSFG, 54% of the GSS and 68% of the GSS Ever Married Catholic, women were married. Those divorced constituted 0.2% of NFP, 7% of NSFG, 12% of GSS and 13% of GSS Ever Married Catholic, while separated women were 0% of NFP, 3% of NSFG, and 4% of both GSS and GSS Ever Married Catholics. NFP respondents had the lowest percentage of cohabitation (0.4%), in comparison to the NSFG (7%) and GSS (7%), and the Ever Married Catholics in the GSS survey with a low rate of 2% had the second lowest percentage. Widows comprised 1% of NFP, 0.5% of NSFG, and 15% of both GSS and GSS Ever Married Catholic groups.

As we observe the marital status of the four groups surveyed, we can't help but wonder whether this curious phenomenon is in great part due to the advantages of the use of Natural Family Planning. The impressive low divorce rate seems to be closely linked to the practice of NFP, but a future matched sample study would enable us to make a more accurate comparison. It cannot be denied that NFP fosters communication and intimate conversation between spouses, as they need to be aware of their combined fertility and infertility. In contrast, it appears that those who have not been given this enrichment have considerably higher divorce, separation and cohabitation rates. Is it possible that a critical element is missing in the marriages of the other groups surveyed? Could the missing element be practicing and sharing the responsibility of Natural Family Planning? Marriages in violation of the Natural Law seem to be in a state of instability due to the lack of chastity within their marriage, resulting in poor communication and cooperation and the denial of mutual responsibility in the area of responsible parenthood.

Figure 7: The Effects of the Sexual Revolution: Advice to a Young Woman or Man regarding way of life.

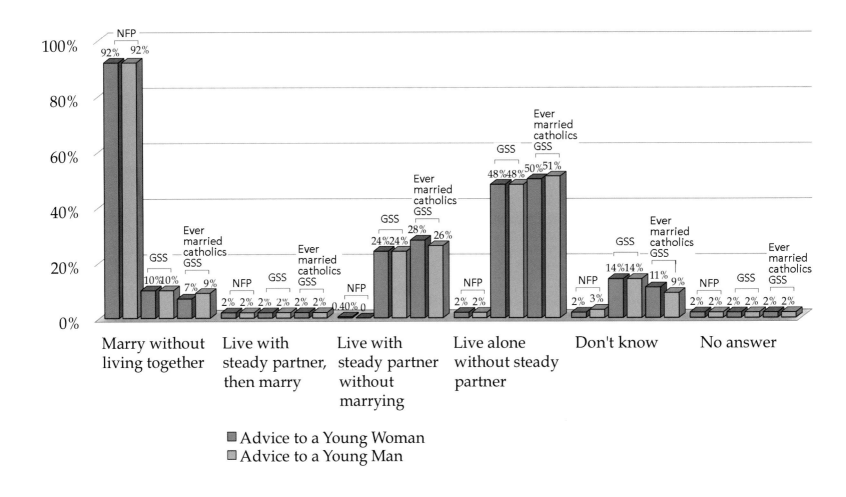

■ Advice to a Young Woman
■ Advice to a Young Man

COMPARATIVE ADJUSTED TABULATIONS

The main objective of this study was to discern if couples who practice NFP are less likely to be divorced than those who do not; so a more direct comparison of groups of similar age and beliefs was necessary.

Adjusted Tabulations

The principal investigator recognized the importance of incorporating adjusted tabulations in the report. This way the NFP sample and the NSFG sample are more directly comparable to each other. It is useful to use some kind of adjustment procedure because the NFP sample consists almost entirely of married Catholics who range in age from 21 to 66 years old, while the NSFG sample consists of women of all faiths including those who have never been married, and who range in age from 15 to 44 years old. These factors: religious affiliation, age, ever married or not, may play a role in accounting for the results obtained thus far.

Therefore, all the adjusted results from the NFP survey are only from those respondents who are Catholic, who have been married at some time in their lives (including those who are currently married), and who range in age from 21 to 44 years old. Similarly, all the adjusted results from the NSFG survey are only from those respondents who are Catholic, who have been married at some time in their lives, (including those who are currently married), and who range in age from 21 to 44 years old. These results are referred to as "adjusted tabulations."

Figure 8: NFP Adjusted and NSFG Adjusted Data - Current Marital Status

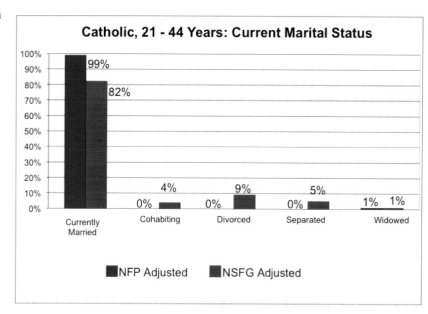

The reason the divorce rate among NFP couples increased from 0.2% to 3% in the adjusted tabulations is because the statistician is using a smaller number of couples in a concentrated age group (21 to 44 years).

Figure 9:

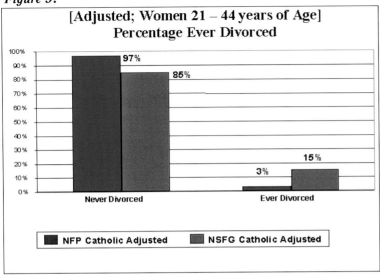

[Adjusted; Women 21 – 44 years of Age]
Percentage Ever Divorced

- 97% Never Divorced (NFP Catholic Adjusted)
- 85% Never Divorced (NSFG Catholic Adjusted)
- 3% Ever Divorced (NFP Catholic Adjusted)
- 15% Ever Divorced (NSFG Catholic Adjusted)

Legend: ■ NFP Catholic Adjusted ■ NSFG Catholic Adjusted

The NFP Catholics who have never divorced is 97%, while the NSFG Catholics who have never divorced is 85%. The divorce rate in the NSFG group increased from 7% to 15% in the adjusted tabulations. The difference between these is 12%, which is a four fold difference.

Figures 8 & 9 provide support for the idea that using NFP among Catholics is associated with family stability. Further research is required in order to determine if this relationship is in any sense causal, or whether the relationship between practicing NFP and family stability is due to other factors common to these couples, including their strong religious beliefs and practices, and whether these developed after they began practicing NFP.

If it is found, after further studies are conducted, that religious fervor is a primary factor in marital stability together with respect for the Natural Law through the practice of NFP, it becomes especially important to prioritize a more faithful adherence to one's chosen faith.

Such findings would provide strong reasons for advocating religious beliefs and practices among the general population who desire a fruitful and lasting marital vocation. If Natural Family Planning is the main reason for the spouse's conversion towards strong religious beliefs and practices, then NFP should be given top priority in all courses that prepare couples for matrimony around the world.

Influences of Intact Families

Unequivocal data has shown that an intact family of a father and a mother has tremendous influence on the behavior of children. Following are some of the findings that show teen pregnancies are influenced by family structure.

Consequences of Family Instability:

- 80% of unintended pregnancies result from contraceptive failure.[9]
- Cohabitations are four times more likely to break up than marriages and less than 4% of cohabitations last 10 years or more.[10]
- The incidence of divorce is 33% to 80% higher among couples who lived together before marriage (this is a good reason to delay the Sacrament of Matrimony until the couple demonstrates that they can live apart while they prepare to accept their mutual fidelity to a fruitful and lasting union).[11]
- Of juveniles and young adults serving time in correctional facilities, 70% come from broken homes.[12]

Figure 10: Facts Concerning Venereal Diseases (VD) [Sexually Transmitted Diseases][13]

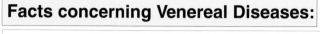

Facts concerning Venereal Diseases:

 Venereal Diseases are the most common diseases in America next to the common cold and flu.

 1 in 5 Americans are presently infected with a Venereal Disease.

 Approximately 19 million new Venereal Disease cases are reported each year.

The direct medical costs for treating Venereal Diseases average $8.4 billion annually.

Benefits of Family Stability:

- Young people aged 14 to 17 who live in a two parent family are less likely to have ever had sexual relations than young people living in any other family arrangement, even after adjusting for potentially confounding factors such as race, age, and socioeconomic deprivation.[14]
- Abstinence and decreased sexual activity among adolescents are primarily responsible for the decline during the 1990's in adolescent pregnancy, birth and abortion rates.[15]
- A three-year program for parents and adolescents promoting family centered human sexuality education accentuating morals and values, lowered teen pregnancies to 1/20th of the national average (5 pregnancies per 1,000 adolescents aged 15 to 19).[16] Since parents are the main influence on their children, they must remain as the primary educators of their children in matters of human sexuality.

Figure 11: NFP, GSS and GSS Ever Married Catholics - Success in Family Life

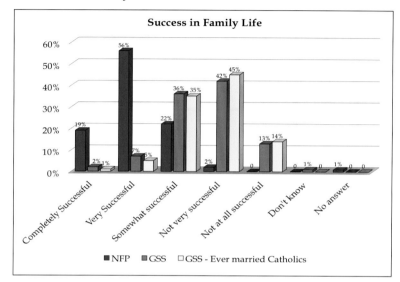

Success in Family Life

A majority of NFP respondents feel successful in family life, while the majority of the GSS and Ever Married Catholics do not. A majority (75%) of NFP respondents feel completely or very successful, and if we also add the "somewhat successful" responses to this, the total becomes 97%. Conversely, only 9% of GSS women and 6% of Ever-Married Catholic women regard themselves as completely or very successful in their family life. If we also add the "somewhat successful" these totals become 45% for GSS and 41% for GSS Ever Married Catholics. The percentage difference is considerable. These responses seem to reflect the vision that to feel successful in family life, it is vital to be faithful and willing to share your most intimate feelings with your spouse, be willing to give to your spouse selflessly without barriers, and to recognize the gift of life and the power to become generous co-creators of new life with God.

ADDITIONAL BENEFITS FROM PRACTICING NFP

Adjusted Comparison of Three Groups

The following information shows a considerable frequency in church attendance among groups #1 & #2 who practice NFP, as compared to group #3 that does not practice NFP:

1. NFP Catholic women aged 21 to 44 years old, married at some time in their life **who practice NFP.**

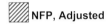 NFP, Adjusted

2. NSFG Catholic women aged 21 to 44 years old, married at some time in their life **who practice NFP.**

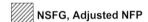 NSFG, Adjusted NFP

3. NSFG Catholic women aged 21 to 44 years old, married at some time in their life **who do not practice NFP.**

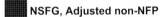 NSFG, Adjusted non-NFP

Figure 12: NFP Adjusted, NSFG Adjusted NFP, NSFG Adjusted non-NFP - Church Attendance

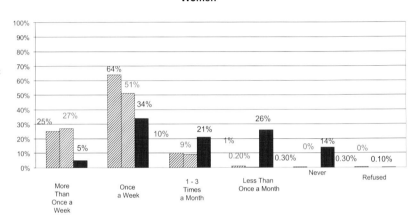

Catholic, 21 - 44 Years: Church Attendance of NFP and non NFP Women

Figure 12 shows the responses of the three groups. Group #1 and #2 have similar responses, which are markedly different from those of group #3. 25% of group #1 and 27% of group #2 attend church more than once a week. In contrast, only 5% of group #3 attend church more than once a week. 64% of group #1 and 51% of group #2 attend church at least once a week, while only 34% of group #3 attend church at least once a week. 0.3% of group #1 and 0% of group #2 never attend church, while 14% of group #3 never attend church. These figures seem to indicate that the importance of prayer and the Sacrament of Matrimony needs to be taught more forcefully in our current culture. It is predictable that those who respect and follow God's Natural Law attain a close relationship with God as they are totally dependent on

His will. Drawing closer to our Creator, in turn, inspires us all the more to observe His laws as they benefit us physically, psychologically, and spiritually.

Conclusions

We have endeavored to show a link between artificial birth control, promiscuity and divorce. The NFP survey respondents: have a dramatically low divorce rate; are happier and more satisfied in their everyday lives; share a deeper intimacy with their spouse; realize a deeper level of communication with their spouse; attend Church more often; and preserve the family unit more responsibly than the other groups. We are thus beginning to demonstrate what has long been asserted philosophically and morally: artificial birth control carries with it a substantial negative impact on the personalistic dimensions of the sexual union of spouses.

"Authentic love is not a vague sentiment or a blind passion. It is an inner attitude that involves the whole human being. It is looking at others, not to use them but to serve them. It is the ability to rejoice with those who are rejoicing and to suffer with those who are suffering. It is sharing what one possesses so that no one may continue to be deprived of what he needs. Love, in a word, is the gift of self…The family, the great workshop of love is the first school, indeed, a lasting school where people are not taught to love with barren ideas, but with incisive power of experience. May every family truly rediscover its own vocation to love. Love that absolutely respects God's plan, love that is the choice and reciprocal gift of self within the family unit."[17]

Endnotes:

[1] Unpublished Study presented at the Medical Committee Meeting of the Knights of Malta, New York, NY 2001.

[2] Dr. Zhang D.W. and J.X. Xu "The Effectiveness of the Ovulation Method" *Reproduction and Contraception*, 1993. Vol.13, No. 3 pp.194-200; Ryder, R.E.J., *British Medical Journal*, Vol. 307, p. 723-726, Sept. 18, 1993.

[3] Arzú Wilson, Mercedes, The Catholic Social Science Review, Vol. VII The Practice of Natural Family Planning vs. the Use of Artificial Birth Control: Family, Sexual and Moral Issues. pp. 185-211, 2002.

[4] Robert T Michael, "Why did the U.S. Divorce Rate Double within a Decade" Research in Population Economics, Vol. 6. p. 367-399. 1988.

[5] William J. Bennett, *"Quantifying Americas Decline"* The Wall Street Journal, March 15, 1993, pp723-726.

[6] Ibid.

[7] Robert T Michael, "Why did the U.S. Divorce Rate Double within a Decade" *Research in Population Economics*, Vol. 6. p. 367-399. 1988.

[8] National Center for Health Statistics. 1996, pp. 367-399.

[9] Trevor Stammers, "Teenage Pregnancies are Influenced by Family Structure" Letters *British Medical Journal*; 324:51, January 5, 2002.

[10] Ibid, cites Morgan P. "Marriage Lite: The rise of Cohabitation and its Consequences" Institute for the Study of Civil Society (CIVITAS): London, 2000:13.

[11] Mercedes Arzú Wilson, Love and Family; Raising a Traditional Family in a Secular World, p. 122; 1996.

[12] Family Research Council, 1996.

[13] Sexual Medical Institute, March 2005. The Alan Guttmacher Inst. May, 2005. American Social Health Association Dec. 1998. Booklet published by the American College of Obstetricians and Gynecologists. Joe S. McIlhaney, Jr., M.D., Safe Sex (Baker Book House, 1991), p. 10.

[14] Trevor Stammers, "Teenage Pregnancies are Influenced by Family Structure" Letters *British Medical Journal*; 324:51, January 5, 2002.

[15] Jeffery Jones M.D. et. al., A Special Report Commissioned by the Consortium of State Physicians Resource Councils, January 7, 1999.

[16] Peggy Kirby and Louis Paradise, "Fertility Appreciation for Families: Evaluation report for the Family of the Americas Foundation" October 1, 1987.

[17] Karol Wojtyla (John Paul II), Love and Responsibility, 1981, p. 42.

X.

Artificial Methods of Birth Control

ARTIFICIAL METHODS OF BIRTH CONTROL

The First "Scientific" Birth Control

Since the early 1930s scientists have known that high doses of androgens, estrogens or progesterone inhibited ovulation. But it would take nearly three more decades before this knowledge would be used to create a method of birth control that could be distributed to the masses.

In 1951 the cofounder of the Worcester Foundation for Experimental Biology (WFEB), Gregory Goodwin Pincus, Ph.D., attended a dinner party where he met birth control supporter Margaret Higgins Sanger, founder of Planned Parenthood. The host of the affair, Abraham Stone, Medical Director and Vice President of the Planned Parenthood Federation of America (PPFA), helped WFEB obtain a grant from PPFA to begin hormonal birth control research. In March 1952 Sanger sent a note to philanthropist Katharine Dexter McCormick in which she mentioned the Foundation's research. An avid birth control advocate, McCormick pledged to increase WFEB's budget to 50 times what it had been with PPFA's grant.

Funding by PPFA and McCormick led to the study of the ovulation-suppressing potential of three oral progestins. Human trials of Enovid, the drug that would be marketed by G.D. Searle & Company, began in Puerto Rico, California and Haiti in April 1956. In June 1957, the U.S. Food and Drug Administration (FDA) approved Enovid for menstrual disorders based on data from its use by more than 600 women.

Diverse Methods of Artificial Birth Control

Today there are many diverse methods of artificial birth control available on the worldwide market. The most commonly used method still comes in pill form. Over the last several decades, three types of birth control pills emerged as the most widely prescribed:

1) a high-dose progestin and estrogen pill, which is no longer widely used due to serious side effects;

2) a low-dose progestin and estrogen ("combination") pill;

3) a progesterone-only ("mini") pill.

The low-dose Combination Pill is now the most prescribed.

Combination Pills

The active ingredients in the combination birth control pill are synthetic versions of estrogen (oestrogen) and a progestin (progestogen). Estrogen and progestin are powerful hormones and a natural part of the female body, but the birth control pill uses them in an unnatural way.

Methods of Operation

Birth control pills have three distinct mechanisms:

1) *May Suppress Ovulation:* A woman ovulates when her pituitary gland, located at the base of the brain, releases hormones that stimulate her ovaries to discharge an ovum (egg). The Combination

Combination Pills

Several additional trials showed Enovid to be a rather effective birth control at the 2.5, 5.0, and 10.0 mg doses. Searle & Company filed a supplemental application with the FDA to add birth control as an approved use for Enovid at the three dose levels. In June 1960 the FDA approved Enovid 10 mg. for birth control. Two years later the 5.0 mg dose was also approved for such use.

In November 1961 it was reported that a woman taking 20 mg. a day of Enavid (the name used for Enovid 10 mg. in the United Kingdom) had developed a blood clot and died. Shortly thereafter two Americans taking Enovid died of thrombosis. By August 1962 the FDA had received reports of 26 women who had developed blood clots. Six of those cases were fatal. Nearly seven years later British scientists conclusively established an elevated risk of venous thrombosis in oral contraceptive users. They also found an increased risk of stroke and myocardial infarction in users who smoke or have high blood pressure or other cardiovascular or cerebrovascular risk factors. Congress responded in the early 1970s merely by requiring drug manufacturers to include a patient package insert with oral contraceptives to address their possible side effects and risks.

Mode of Action of the Pill, the Patch, Implants, NuvaRing, and Depo-Provera Injection

1. Inhibits Ovulation

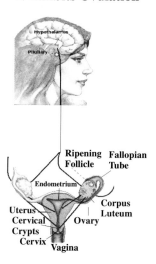

1. The high levels of estrogen and progestin may suppress the 2 hormones FSH and LH and prevent them from being released by the pituitary gland in the brain thus inhibiting ovulation.

2. Thickens the Cervical Mucus

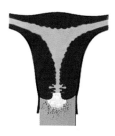

2. The levels of progestin may thicken the cervical mucus making sperm migration difficult.

3. Prevents the normal build up of the endometrium

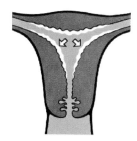

3. Doesn't allow the normal buildup of the endometrial lining of the woman's uterus. Thus, if conception occured, the newly conceived baby tries to implant but does not find enough nourishment to remain in the uterus for the rest of the pregnancy. This is the abortificient effect of the methods.

Pill may interrupt the release of these pituitary hormones, preventing the ovaries from releasing an ovum. Without an ovum available for conception, a woman has been essentially rendered chemically sterile.

2) *May Impede Sperm Migration:* Before a woman ovulates her cervix produces mucus through which sperm migrate to meet the ovum. The mucus also provides nourishment to sustain the life of the sperm. When a woman is under the influence of progestin the mucus thickens, which impedes sperm migration.

3) *May Inhibit Implantation:* If the Pill fails to prevent pregnancy with one of the first two actions, the union of the ovum with the sperm (conception) will result in the creation of human life. Five to six days later this new human being will attempt to implant in the endometrium (the lining of the uterus). The progestin component of the combination and mini pill causes the lining of the uterus to be thin, which makes it inhospitable to the newly conceived life. This leads to a chemically-induced miscarriage (abortion).

Any one of these three mechanism will achieve the desired result. A woman taking a Combined Oral Contraceptive will not know which one of the three mechanisms worked.

Cancer

The risk of cancer has long been a primary worry associated with the use of birth control pills:

- Pill users have a significantly higher risk of developing a precancerous condition of the cervix (cervical displasia, which exposes the most vulnerable cells to the human papilloma virus (HPV)).
- The risk of cervical cancer has nearly quadrupled for women infected with HPV and who use the Pill for five or more years.

- Low dose pills have been associated with greater breast cancer risk compared to high-dose regimens. This could be due to the more potent progestin used in the newer drugs.
- A woman who ingests combined oral contraceptives before her first full-term pregnancy increases her risk of developing pre-menopause breast cancer by 44%.
- A woman taking the Pill for at least four years prior to her first full-term pregnancy has a 52% increased chance of developing breast cancer.
- Studies have shown that long-time users have an increased risk of developing liver tumors. Drug manufacturers describe the tumors as "typically benign" (as opposed to "always benign"), but it is noted that such a tumor could cause "fatal internal bleeding" if it were to rupture.

In 2005 the World Health Organization classified combined oral contraceptives as a Group I carcinogen (the most dangerous).

Sexually Transmitted Diseases

In 2006 the U.S. Centers for Disease Control and Prevention (CDC) reported that the use of combined oral contraceptives is associated with cervical Chlamydia. If not treated, the infection can result in female sterility.

An individual infected with a sexually transmitted disease is up to five times more likely than an uninfected person to contract the human immunodeficiency virus (HIV) if exposed through sexual contact. Furthermore, an individual infected with HIV who also has another sexually transmitted disease is more likely to transmit HIV through sexual contact than other HIV-infected persons. HIV may lead to acquired immunodeficiency syndrome (AIDS).

Menstrual Bleeding

Research has demonstrated that the Combination Pill poses the risk of unhealthy changes in menstrual bleeding. Bleeding irregularities are most likely during the first three months of use. After discontinuing the Pill, some women may experience infrequent, very light or no menstrual periods. This generally happens when such a condition was pre-existent and may result in difficulty in conceiving.

Drug Failure

Women who become pregnant while on the birth control pill may face serious problems:

- If the birth control pill fails, an ectopic pregnancy may occur. In an ectopic pregnancy a new human life has implanted outside the uterus. 95% of ectopic pregnancies occur in the fallopian tubes, but an ovum may also implant in the ovary, abdomen or cervix. Since these areas hold neither the required nurturing tissue nor adequate space, the affected organ will eventually burst, which will result in the death of the baby and endanger the life of the mother.
- There is an increase in congenital problems and gender ambiguity in children whose mothers become pregnant while taking the Pill or within six months after discontinuing it.
- Birth control hormones cause a folic acid deficiency, especially in women with poor nutritional intake and/or those who used the Pill for a long period of time. Folic acid deficiency is related to neural tube defects such as spina bifida (some vertebrae overlying the spinal cord are not fully formed and remain unfused and open) and anencephaly (the forebrain, the largest part of the brain, is missing).

Other Adverse Effects

Women taking the birth control pill face many increased risks, some of which are serious and may even cause death:

- heart attack (when there are other factors present such as high blood pressure or smoking)
- stroke (when there are other factors present such as high blood pressure or smoking)
- fluid retention (may lead to high blood pressure)
- blood clots
- varicose veins
- breast tenderness or pain
- gallbladder disease
- decreased libido
- migraine headaches
- mood swings
- nausea or vomiting
- decreased quantity and quality of breast milk
- vision problems (when using contact lens)
- weight gain
- benign liver tumors that may cause death if they rupture (due to internal abdominal bleeding)

Progestin-Only Pills (Mini-Pills)

"Progestin-only" is something of a misnomer. Mini-Pills do not actually contain progesterone, but one of several chemically related compounds in many different formulations. Unlike Combination Pills, however, Mini-Pills do not contain estrogen.

The Mini-Pill must be taken every 24 hours, which means there are no hormone-free days. It is successful in suppressing ovulation only about 50% of the time, although makers have recently claimed it does so "most of the time." Mini-Pills thicken the cervical mucus which may impede migrating sperm. The primary mechanism of action is the thinning of the endometrium to inhibit implantation, resulting in an abortion.

There are currently six brands of the Mini-Pill on the international market, but none are available in every country of the world: Cerazette, Femulen, Micronor/Micro-Novom, Norgeston, and Noriday/Locilan.

Brand Name	Key Ingredient	Manufacturer	Availability
Cerazette	desogestrel	Organon (Merck & Company)	Africa, Europe, Latin America
Femulen	etynodiol diacetate	Pharmacia (Pfizer)	Africa, Asia, Australia, Europe
Micronor/Micro-Novom	norethisterone	Janssen-Cilag (Johnson & Johnsn)	Africa, Australia, Latin America, North America
Norgeston	levonorgestrel	Schering Health Care (Merck & Company)	Europe, North America
Noriday/Locilan	norethisterone	Pfizer	Australia, Europe

Adverse Effects

Several problems have been linked to the Mini-Pill:

- increased risk of developing breast cancer
- irregular periods ranging from no menstrual periods to increased days of spotting and bleeding
- ectopic pregnancy
- skin spots
- breast tenderness
- ovarian cysts
- nausea
- headache
- dizziness
- depression, anxiety, irritability
- weight change
- fatigue
- increased cholesterol

It is important to note that long-term effects of combined oral birth control have been studied over 50 years, but research into long-term effects of newer methods of birth control, including the Mini-Pill, is relatively scarce. Therefore, it is likely that unsuspected side-effects, some of which could be serious, will eventually come to light.

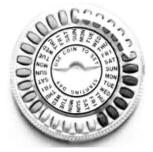

The Patch (Ortho-Evra)

Ortho-Evra is a transdermal patch that releases synthetic estrogen (ethinyl estradiol) and progestin (norelgestromin) hormones. In the United States, Ortho-Evra is marketed by Ortho-McNeil. In Canada the product is called Evra and is marketed by Janssen-Ortho. In the United Kingdom and other parts of the world it is marketed by Janssen-Cilag. All three companies are divisions of Johnson & Johnson. Ortho-Evra/Evra is the only birth control patch currently on the market.

The square patch is applied to the skin on the upper arm, buttocks, abdomen or thigh. The mode of action is the same as the Pill. Women who use The Patch, however, are exposed to 60% more estrogen than those ingesting a birth control pill.

Adverse Effects

Side effects of The Patch are similar to those reported by users of the birth control pill.

More specifically related to The Patch are some significantly more adverse effects:

- The Patch has been linked to a doubled risk of blood clots because of its increased estrogen dose. Patient reports between 2002 and 2004 showed The Patch to be 12 times more likely to cause strokes and 18 times more likely to cause blood clots than the conventional birth control pill. By 2007 at least 1,500 lawsuits and 23 deaths had been linked to its use.
- Some users had complaints related to the application site, including partial or complete detachment.
- Darkening and irritation of the skin has been reported.
- Some women experienced nausea.
- Women have reported breast discomfort or pain.
- Some women suffered from headaches.
- The Patch has been shown to be less effective in women who weigh more than 198 pounds.

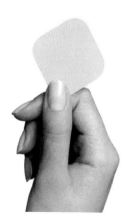

Vaginal Ring (NuvaRing)

The Vaginal Ring is a flexible, soft ring made of plastic that contains estrogen (ethinyl estradiol) and progestin (etonogestrel). It is kept in place for 21 days and removed for seven days. Its mode of action is similar to the Pill.

Adverse Effects

The Vaginal Ring carries the health complications possible with all combined hormonal birth control. Several more potentially serious problems have been linked specifically to the Vaginal Ring:

- vaginal discomfort, vaginal discharge, vaginitis
- headaches
- nausea
- tenderness of the breasts
- blotchy, dark areas on the skin (melasma)

It should be noted that 15.1% of women stopped using the Vaginal Ring due to adverse effects such as experiencing the sensation of the existence of a foreign body, emotional issues, weight gain, coital problems and expulsion. Furthermore, if the Vaginal Ring affixes to vaginal tissue only a healthcare professional should remove it.

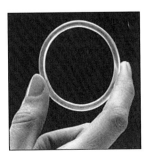

Implant (Implanon)

The pursuit of a subcutaneous birth control implant began in 1966. Development was made possible by the discovery of silicone and its biocompatibility with the human body. This technology later resulted in the development of Norplant and Jadelle (Norplant-2).

The Implant has silastic tubes with sealed ends that provide a sustained release of steroids over several months. The first implant to reach the market was Norplant. It consisted of six rods containing a progestin (levonorgestrel). It was placed under the skin in the upper arm, which required a local anesthetic, and was said to be effective for five years.

Norplant was initially marketed outside of the United States beginning in 1983. It was approved by the FDA in 1990 and became available the following year. Norplant was withdrawn from the UK market in 1999 and its U.S. distributor, Wyeth Inc. (now part of Pfizer Inc.), announced in 2002 that it would no longer make Norplant available in the United States. However, it is still used in the developing world. In the United Kingdom, Norplant has been replaced by Nexplanon, which is also manufactured by Pfizer. Nexplanon must be removed after three years.

Jadelle, also known as Norplant-2, was intended to be a replacement for Norplant. Approved by the FDA in 1996, it is a 2-rod system which, like its predecessor, contains levonorgestrel. Despite FDA approval, Jadelle has not been marketed in the United States, but it is used in other countries.

Implanon, a single-rod implant containing etonogestrel that is said to be effective for three years, entered the international market in 1998. It was approved by the FDA in 2006 and is currently the only birth control implant available in the United States. Implanon was developed by Organon International. The company was purchased by Schering-Plough Corporation in 2007. Two years later Schering-Plough merged with Merck & Company (known as Merck Sharp & Dohme outside the United States and Canada).

Adverse Effects

Many complications have been associated with Implanon, including:

- problems with implant insertion, including incomplete insertions and/or infections which may lead to expulsion
- difficulty in removing the device when the implant is too deep, not palpable, encased in fibrous tissue or has migrated to other parts of the body
- decreased local sensibility
- changes in menstrual bleeding (irregular, heavier or lighter, more or less frequent, continuous or prolonged, or stopped altogether)
- headache
- acne
- weight gain or loss
- breast tenderness or pain
- irritation, bruising, rash, pain, itching, scarring and/or abscess at site of implant
- fatigue
- increased appetite
- depression, mood swings, nervousness, anxiety
- decreased libido
- dizziness
- hot flushes
- flatulence
- ovarian cysts
- difficulty sleeping

- sleepiness
- vomiting
- constipation, diarrhea
- hair growth on face and body, hair loss
- vaginal discharge, itching
- aching muscles and/or joints
- breast enlargement
- fluid retention
- rise in blood pressure
- breast cancer
- thrombosis (blood clot), including pulmonary embolism, blindness, and stroke
- yellowing of the skin or eyes (jaundice)
- sudden severe abdominal pain
- bleeding
- infections
- influenza-like symptoms, feeling sick, nausea
- ectopic pregnancies
- migraine headaches (in 25% of users)
- trouble using contact lenses, and
- spotty darkening of the skin, especially on the face

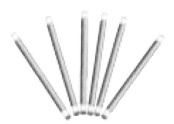 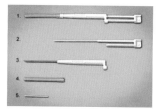

Nexplanon

The newly introduced implant on the market.

Nexplanon is removed in the same way as Implanon.

Implanon (etonogestrel) has been replaced by Nexplanon. The new version of the contraceptive implant is bioequivalent to Implanon and is removed in the same way. However, it contains barium to allow localization on X-ray or CT scan.

It is obvious that the manufacturers have been losing implants in different parts of the woman's body making it essential for this new version to contain an additional foreign chemical. Barium is necessary in order to "track" the location of the implant that has traveled somewhere else in her body, making it easier for medical professionals to do an X-ray or CT scan to find it.

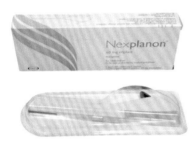

I wonder if governments will make it mandatory for the manufacturers of these new implants to provide X-ray and CT scan equipment in towns and villages throughout the Third World where implants are being inserted without warnings or professional medical care.

There is no reason to believe that Nexplanon will not have the same serious side effects as its two predecessors, Norplant and Implanon.

The Injection (Depo-Provera)

Injectable birth control is administered into a muscle of the body (thigh, buttocks, or deltoid) every 11 to 13 weeks. It contains progesterone (depot medroxyprogesterone acetate). Depo-Provera is the brand name for a 150 mg aqueous injection. It was approved by the FDA in December 2004. Depo-subQ Provera 104 is a variation of the original Depo-Provera that is instead 104 mg that is placed under the skin. It contains 69% of progesterone found in the original drug. Depo-Provera and Depo-subQ Provera 104 are manufactured by Pfizer Inc.

Adverse Effects

Depo-Provera has been one of the most risky forms of birth control ever approved for use in the United States. Its potential side effects include:

- decreased libido
- depression
- breast tenderness
- increases risk of contracting sexually transmitted diseases
- pain or discomfort
- weight gain
- headache
- asthenia (weakness or fatigue)
- no hair growth or hair loss (alopecia)
- nervousness
- delayed return of fertility (up to 12 months after last injection)
- there is a greater loss of memory among women who ever used Depo-Provera

- breast cancer (as high as 190% of young women who used Depo-Provera for three years or longer)
- low birth weight and an 80% greater chance of dying in the first year of life for infants exposed to Depo-Provera while in the womb
- increase in chromosomal anomalies and birth defects such as masculinization of the external genitalia of females
- results in early demineralization of a women's bones even before menopause

Depo-Provera and Menstrual Bleeding

In addition, Depo-Provera can affect menstrual bleeding. After one year of use, 55% of women experienced amenorrhea. After two years of use the rate rose to 68%. In the first months of use "irregular or unpredictable bleeding or spotting, or rarely, heavy or continuous bleeding" was reported.

Depo-Provera and Bone Loss

A few more words about the relationship between Depo-Provera and bone loss are in order. It has long been known that Depo-Provera causes bone loss but only recently has it been discovered that the osteoporotic effects of the injection grow worse the longer Depo-Provera is administered. Moreover, the effects can remain long after the injections are stopped and may even be irreversible. In November 2004 the FDA and Pfizer agreed to place a "black box warning" on the Depo-Provera label. The FDA and Pfizer recommend that Depo-Provera not be used for longer than two years, unless there is no viable alternative method of contraception, due to concerns over bone loss.

Depo-Provera - Black Box Warning

When the U.S. Congress learned of the significant health risks associated with the first birth control pill it merely required that the manufacturer develop a product information insert. In the case of Depo-Provera, the required "black box warning" appears on the package insert for prescription drugs "that may cause serious adverse effects." A black box warning indicates that medical studies have shown that the drug carries a "significant risk of serious or even life-threatening adverse effects." The FDA can require a pharmaceutical company to place a black box warning on the label of any prescription drug, or in literature describing it. It is the strongest warning the FDA can require.

The Health of Women in Jeopardy

The FDA and Pfizer continue to let women use Depo-Provera if "there is no viable alternative method of contraception." It gets worse. According to the World Health Organization, a division of the United Nations, use of Depo-Provera should not be restricted. And in 2008 a committee of the American College of Obstetricians and Gynecologists told healthcare providers that concerns about bone mineral density loss "should neither prevent the prescription of nor continuation of Depo-Provera beyond two years of use." Some have suggested that when birth control is the subject, politics and profits trump scientific studies and the health of women.

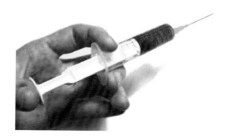

Intrauterine Device

The intrauterine device (IUD) is a small T-shaped gadget with an attached string. It is inserted inside the uterus through the cervical canal. There are two types of IUDs currently on the market. The first releases copper that is toxic to cells and causes a chronic inflammation of the endometrium. The second releases a progestin that alters the development of the endometrium.

In each menstrual cycle the womb builds up tissue and chemical substances that help the survival and movement of the sperm in order to maintain a favorable environment for implantation (the process through which a new embryo unites with the womb to obtain nutrition to survive). In contrast, all IUDs weaken and cause a chronic inflammation of the endometrium because they contain trace metals or hormones. This impedes the implantation of newly conceived human life. The copper IUD damages the ovum or kills sperm through the toxic effect of the copper. This toxicity can also damage or destroy an embryo.

The Mirena hormonal IUD can reduce the likelihood of ovulation in about 15% of cycles. It can turn cervical mucus into a thick, sticky substance which reduces the possibility of sperm penetration. The IUD releases a synthetic progestin, which alters the development of the endometrium, thereby making it hostile to the implantation of the baby in the womb.

Nearly 50% of women discontinue use of the IUD due to its serious side effects. Women of poor health in the developing world have an even higher discontinuation rate because they are already weak, anemic and unable to tolerate the severe and prolonged hemorrhages caused by the IUD's abortifacient effect.

Adverse Effects

Research has tied the IUD to several health problems:

- Pregnancy with an IUD in place may cause severe infection, shock, miscarriage, premature labor or death.
- There is an increased risk of ectopic pregnancy.
- The abortifacient effect causes heavier and longer menstrual periods, as well as spotting between periods. (Normal menstruation disappears in 20% of hormonal IUD users.)
- IUD users are susceptible to Pelvic Inflammatory Disease, which causes pelvic pain, heavy bleeding, fever, and fallopian tube damage. This can result in permanent sterility.
- An IUD may embed in the uterus, which could make it difficult to remove.
- Perforation may occur. Breastfeeding mothers have a higher rate of perforation.
- Ovarian cysts occur in 12% of hormonal IUD users.
- A variety of vaginal infections, including Candida, are caused by the string attached to the IUD that acts as a ladder for bacteria to enter the womb.
- Severe anemia, menstrual cramps, backache, joint aches, and vaginal discharge may occur.
- Up to 10% of the time the body will reject the IUD without the woman being aware of it. If this occurs once, there is a 30% chance it will happen again. An IUD may also be spontaneously expelled from the vagina.
- There have been reported cases of toxic shock syndrome, staphylococcus aureus, squamous cell carcinoma (cancer of the bladder), tumors and abscesses.

The most serious consequence of using the IUD is its abortifacient effect. A woman with an IUD in her womb may unknowingly have as many as 1.8 abortions per year.

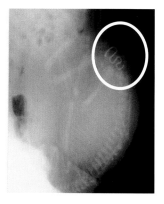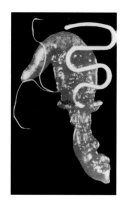

Left: X-ray of a baby about to be born with an IUD implanted in his back. Right: IUD that perforated a uterus and was found in the woman's appendix.

The baby tries to implant in spite of the IUD and struggles to survive; due to constant inflammation the baby cannot receive the normal nourishment and an abortion takes place.

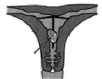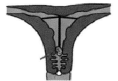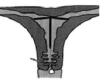

The baby implants in spite of the IUD. As baby grows the danger of the IUD rupturing the amniotic sac increases. It is a very dangerous pregnancy.

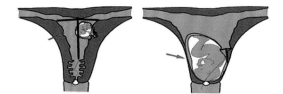

"Emergency Contraception"

"Emergency contraception" refers to a group of drugs and devices that prevent implantation of a newly conceived human life, thereby causing an abortion. To this end, women are encouraged to use pills and devices to prevent pregnancy right after the sexual act has taken place.

Effectiveness

It is very difficult to measure the efficacy of "emergency contraception" because a woman is fertile only for about 100 hours in her menstrual cycle and most women are not aware of their fertile time. "Emergency contraception" will come down in history as the most dangerous drug given to young girls whose bodies are still developing. No study has demonstrated that the increase of access to these dangerous synthetic chemicals has reduced the *pregnancy* rate.

"Morning After Pill"

The "morning after pill" is a phrase used to describe a group of drugs taken after intercourse in order to prevent pregnancy. Some "morning after pills" contain only synthetic progesterone and others are a combination of synthetic estrogen and progesterone. These pills contain large doses of the same synthetic chemicals found in the birth control pill, therefore, women will experience the same serious side effects as the birth control pill.

The "New 'Morning After Pill'"

"Ella" (ulipristal acetate) has been introduced as the "new morning after pill." It blocks the effects of progesterone in the uterine lining by not allowing the normal growth of the endometrium, thereby preventing implantation. It can be taken up to five days after intercourse because of its abortifacient effect. "Ella" was approved by the FDA in August 2010.

"Mifepristone (RU-486)"

A well known abortifacient pill, Mifepristone blocks the effect of progesterone, the hormone that is vital to support pregnancy as it maintains the endometrium, where the embryo implants. When deprived of oxygen and its source of nutrition, the baby dies. Mifepristone is administered with a prostaglandin that causes contractions of the uterus, (to expel the baby).

Adverse effects of this abortifacient drug include serious blood loss, pain that may require narcotics, vomiting, diarrhea, fever, nausea, fatigue, bronchospasm, and excessive thirst. In addition, several birth defects (scalp, cranium and limb abnormalities) have been linked to Mifepristone and prostaglandin.

"Copper-T"

The Copper-T IUD is sometimes used as an emergency contraception device. It affects the normal growth of the lining of the uterus in order to prevent implantation of the newly conceived baby, therefore acting as an abortifacient.

Prophylactics (Condoms)

Condoms are usually made of latex, but some are made from polyurethane, polyisoprene, or lamb intestine. The female condom is most often made of nitrile. Condoms are not particularly effective in preventing pregnancy. A woman can conceive during only about 100 hours of her menstrual cycle, but sexually transmitted diseases (syphilis, gonorrhea, HPV, Chlamydia, and so forth) may be transmitted every day of the year.

Deterioration

When condoms are not stored in a fresh and dry place they deteriorate, which limits the time of effectiveness because the materials deteriorate. The use of lubricants and spermicides can make condoms fail because they accelerate damage.

Statistical Effectiveness

Condoms are effective in preventing pregnancy some 84-88% of the time. (The chance of pregnancy over one year of use is one in six.) The pregnancy rate for girls (under the age of 18) where condoms were used is 18.4%. Unmarried minority women using condoms had a pregnancy rate of up to 36%. Unmarried Hispanic women had a 44.5% pregnancy rate.

Condoms Do Not Protect Against HIV

Claims that condoms can be an effective means of preventing the spread of HIV, which can lead to AIDS, are false. After a great deal of research, health authorities in the United States concluded that some methods of birth control, including condoms, increase the risk of becoming infected with HIV. This is due to a chemical component that decreases the capacity of the immunological system. Furthermore, HIV is 500 times smaller than a human sperm. Since condoms fail to prevent pregnancy anywhere from 12 to 44% of the time, they are far less effective in preventing the transmission of this tiny virus.

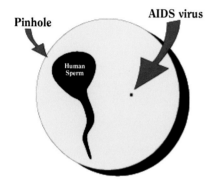

Condom Failure Around the World

United States: In 2005, 96% of public schools in the State of California implemented an aggressive "sex education" program promoting the use of condoms. Despite this program, over one million youngsters in California, or one out of every four, have a sexually transmitted disease.

Botswana: Following the recommendations of international "experts", The Republic of Botswana promoted condom use and distributed antiviral drugs in a nationwide effort to curb the spread of HIV. Despite a condom promotional campaign costing US $13.5 million, about 25% of the population is currently infected with HIV. The use of condoms

and those infected with HIV have increased at the same rate and are the highest of any country in Africa.

Uganda: In contrast, "Education for Life" is a program that encourages young people to remain virgins until marriage and to stay faithful within marriage. Developed by Sister Doctor Mirian Duggan with support from the government of the Republic of Uganda, participants are educated about the physical and moral consequences of sexual promiscuity. "Education for Life" has significantly reduced the spread of sexually transmitted diseases. In January 2004, a meeting of international experts agreed that "the most effective way to avoid infection is going back to abstinence and mutual fidelity among noninfected persons."

"We cannot associate a greater use of condoms with a lesser rate of AIDS...," said Edward C. Green, Ph.D., senior research scientist at the Harvard School of Public Health, and director of the AIDS Prevention Research Project at the Harvard University Center for Population and Development Studies. "Our best studies show a consistent relationship between more availability of condoms and an increase (not a decrease) of AIDS infections...Our research shows that the reduction in the number of sexual partners is the most important behavioral change linked to the decrease of infection."

UNAIDS, a United Nations program on HIV/AIDS, asked Dr. Norman Hearst, an epidemiologist at the University of California at San Francisco, to scientifically prove that condom distribution had curbed the spread of HIV. But Norman found that the greater number of condoms per person, the greater the number of HIV/AIDS cases.

It should be remembered that condoms constitute only a limited measure of efficacy. When it is said that condoms make sexual behavior "safe" there is a risk that the population will engage in increasingly risky behaviors. Such behaviors create bad habits that can eventually make useless any claims of preventive efficacy.

Thailand: In 1991 the Kingdom of Thailand implemented measures designed to fight the spread of HIV. The government's Minister of Health approved a program promoting "100% use of condoms." All homes were encouraged to have a supply of condoms on hand and condom vending machines were installed in supermarkets, restaurants, bars and other public places. This program was widely accepted by the people.

Philippines: In contrast, in 1993 René Bullecer, M.D., received authorization from the Catholic Bishops Conference in the Philippines to establish "Free of AIDS," which became the country's official program against HIV/AIDS. The government of the Republic of the Philippines supported the program. By the end of 2003 the disparity in the efficacy of both programs was evident (see table).

Parameter	Thailand	Philippines
Population	62,833,000	79,999,000
AIDS--Related Deaths in 2003	58,000	500
Adults & Children with HIV	570,000	9,000
HIV Infection Rate	9,072,000	113,000

This table shows that the HIV Rate in Thailand is 80 times higher than in the Philippines, which is due to tradition and religion. In the Philippines they do not promote promiscuity *and* married persons remain faithful to their spouses.

Reaching Youth

It is critical that young people be motivated to value abstinence before marriage and fidelity thereafter. It is the only way to preserve their health and wellbeing, as well as their spouse's and the children they will have.

In Latin America condom use has been encouraged. Yet this approach has resulted in dismal failure. It would be better to imitate the many African countries (Lesotho, Malawi, Mozambique, Namibia, South Africa, Tanzania, Zambia, and Zimbabwe) that have established a campaign under the motto "Only One Love." In effect since October 2008, this program encourages monogamy and fidelity as a measure against the spread of HIV; precisely because it has been proven that it is the most effective way to decrease the chance of being infected with a sexually transmitted disease.

Sterilization

The fallopian tubes are two important organs located below the abdomen and connected to the uterus. They help in the transportation of sperm to the ovum and when conception takes place their hair-like cilia reverses direction to transport the newly conceived baby to implant in the uterus. This natural process takes approximately five to six days.

Tubal Ligation

Tubal ligation is the only surgical procedure that renders healthy organs dysfunctional. It is a birth control method that requires tying, cutting, burning or blocking the fallopian tubes to disrupt movement of the ovum to the uterus and sperm from traveling to the ovum.

The two most common procedures are laparoscopy (abdomen is inflated with carbon dioxide, a fiber optic cable system is introduced through a small incision, surgical instruments are inserted to cut, tie or burn the tubes) and minilaparotomy (an incision is made in the abdomen and the fallopian tubes are closed with clips, burned, cut and tied).

While often passed off as completely safe, tubal ligation has been associated with several significant problems:

- Tubal ligation requires the administration of anesthesia, which carries its own set of risks.
- It is not 100% effective as pregnancy can still occur up to 5.4% of the time.
- In the long-term, there is a 5% to 25% increased risk of heavy menses.
- Increased risk of pelvic pain.
- Tubal ligation may cause depression and anxiety.
- Within 14 years of getting a tubal ligation, nearly 17% of women need a hysterectomy.
- There can be a decrease in sexual desire.
- Women who undergo a tubal ligation may develop premature ovarian failure, which can result in irregular or missed periods, hot flashes, night sweats, vaginal dryness, irritability and/or difficulty concentrating.

Women who undergo a tubal ligation may develop post tubal ligation syndrome (PTLS). Due to conflicting study results, many doctors do not recognize the existence of PTLS, but an increasing number of medical professionals and women who had their tubes tied, are convinced that the syndrome is real. In fact, in recent years there has been a significant increase in the number of support groups and websites that specifically address PTLS. Whether recognized by any one person in medicine or not, the fact remains that many women are suffering from long-term problems they did not have before their tubal ligation.

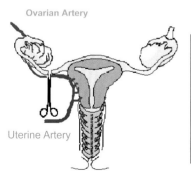

In 56% of women the ovary receives blood from the ovarian and uterine arteries.

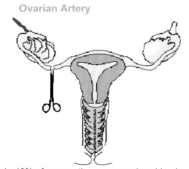

In 40% of women the ovary receives blood only from the ovarian artery.

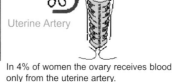

In 4% of women the ovary receives blood only from the uterine artery.

One website that addresses PTLS noted the failure of some doctors to recognize the condition.

When speaking with their physicians and describing the various symptoms taking place, women are often given the following answers, none of which mentions treatment or cure:

- "You are just getting older and your body is changing."
- "Nothing changes with your body after a tubal ligation."
- "Post Tubal Ligation Syndrome does not exist."
- "It's all in your head and maybe you are depressed. We will prescribe an anti-depressant for you."

Walking away frustrated and humiliated, these women know this is not in their heads and they need to find out if there is a cure. They do not want to live with the symptoms plaguing them and they want their health back.

There are several symptoms associated with PTLS, the most common being severe cramps, increased menstrual pain, bleeding, and premenstrual tension. But many other problems are associated with the procedure:

- ectopic pregnancy or pregnancies
- hot flashes, flushes, night sweats and/or cold flashes, clammy feeling, chills
- bouts of rapid heart beat
- irritability, anxiety, mood swings, depression, sudden tears, feeling ill at ease, dread, apprehension, doom
- trouble sleeping (with or without night sweats)
- irregular periods (shorter, longer, lighter, heavier)
- loss of libido
- itchy vagina—at times raw-like, can radiate from whole area, even with absence of yeast infections
- crashing fatigue

- difficulty concentrating, disorientation, mental confusion, memory lapses
- incontinence
- prolapsed uterus due to rapid decrease in estrogen levels
- itchy, crawly skin
- aching or sore joints, muscles and tendons
- increased tension in muscles
- breast tenderness
- decrease in breast mass
- headache change: increase or decrease
- gastrointestinal distress, indigestion, flatulence, gas pain, nausea
- sudden bouts of bloat
- exacerbation of existing conditions
- increase in allergies
- weight gain
- hair loss or thinning hair (head, pubic, or whole body) and/or increase in facial hair
- dizziness, light-headedness, episodes of loss of balance
- changes in body odor
- electric "shock" or "stabbing" sensation under the skin
- tingling in the extremities
- gum bleeding, burning tongue, burning roof of mouth, bad taste in mouth, change in breath odor
- osteoporosis (after several years)
- changes in fingernails (softer, crack or break easier)

Many women have reported that they simultaneously suffered from more than half of the aforesaid symptoms.

One expert on PTLS has said that a primary reason why it is not recognized as a true syndrome by many doctors is that "there is no specific diagnostic test that is correlated with symptoms."

Essure: A New Non-surgical Sterilization Procedure

There is a new permanent sterilization method available in the United States. Essure involves the placement of micro-inserts in the fallopian tubes to form scar tissue. In this procedure, called hysteroscopy, a micro-insert is introduced through the vagina, the cervix and the uterus. It is then placed in each of the fallopian tubes. After the procedure, the body and the micro-insert function together to form a barrier of tissue that prevents sperm from reaching the ovum. It takes three to six months for the tissue to grow and form a permanent scar.

There are two primary side effects associated with Essure:
1) infection, and 2) tubal perforation. It is important to remember, however, that this is a relatively new procedure that is technically in its "introductory phase." Long-term effectiveness and potential consequences have not yet been evaluated, which means the women who undergo the procedure are essentially serving as the manufacturer's "guinea pigs."

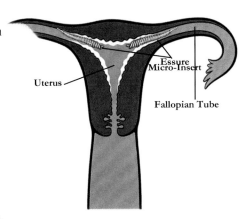

Female Sterilization Reversal

Many women who have been sterilized feel the desire to restore their fertility. Some have remarried and wish to have a child with their new husband. Others feel the need to recover their physical integrity or some feel they have done something immoral and wish to obtain spiritual healing. But significant obstacles exist for those wishing to reverse sterilization. For example, surgery is more extensive and expensive than the original procedure because they are not generally covered by health insurance. The return to fertility is never guaranteed. The overall success rate varies depending on the age of the woman, the kind of sterilization technique employed, and the surgeon's expertise.

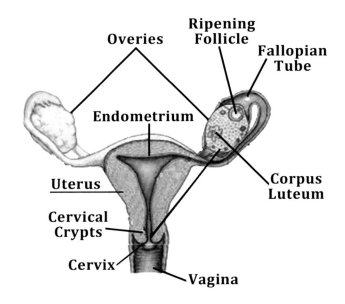

Summary of the Normal Male Reproductive System

Sperm are produced, stored, and delivered by the male reproductive system. The male reproductive physiology includes the testes, urethra, vas deferens, prostate gland, seminal vesicle, and penis.

Immature sperm migrate from the seminiferous tubules to the epididymis to mature and be stored. The mature sperm travel from the epididymis through the vas deferens. The vas deferens is a narrow, muscular tube about 18 inches long. Its smooth muscle contractions propel the sperm forward. They arrive first at the widest part of the vas deferens, and then pass into the ejaculatory ducts. In the ejaculatory ducts, a liquid secretion from the seminal vesicles mixes with the sperm. Semial fluid contains fructose sugar, which the sperm use as fuel.

The liquid mixture is propelled forward through the ejaculatory ducts toward the urethra, passing first through the prostate gland, where milky prostatic fluid is added, forming the substance we call semen. The prostatic lid helps the sperm swim faster, which is important for getting to the egg cell.

Finally, about a teaspoon of semen is ejected out (ejaculated) through the far end of the urethra at the end of the penis. From the time the sperm leave the man's body, they have between 12 and 48 hours to find the egg cell, assuming an egg is available. Of the 300 to 400 million sperm ejaculated, only about 200 or so will survive to reach the egg cell and usually, only one will succeed in conceiving a new human life.

Vasectomy

Vasectomy is a surgery intended to permanently sterilize a man by a surgical procedure in which the ducts that carry sperm out of the testes are cut and tied off so that no sperm can pass. Vasectomy is a form of male sterilization and is used as a method of birth control. The procedure has no effect on a man's capacity to produce semen; the only difference is that his semen will no longer contain sperm. Semen is a cloudy white fluid primarily made up of secretions from male reproductive organs. Semen serves to nourish and "transport" sperm to the vagina. Sperm normally enters semen at sexual climax via the vas deferens (thin tubes in the scrotum). A vasectomy prevents sperm from releasing into semen because the vas deferens is cut and sealed, which essentially blocks the "road" sperm would have needed to travel to meet up with the semen. When the sperm channel is interrupted in such a way, a man becomes surgically sterile.

The body continues to produce sperm after a vasectomy just as it did before the procedure. The sperm is absorbed by the body, which may cause the immune system to recognize the cells as foreign proteins. To fight the foreign invaders, the body produces antibodies. This occurs in as many as 80% of men who have a vasectomy. Immune reactions can also cause arteries to clog, which in turn could cause a heart attack.

A vasectomy patient may experience chronic orchialagia. This is a dull post-vasectomy pain or ache in the testicles that is thought to be caused by a congestion of the epididymis which has filled with dead sperm and fluid.

New Research at Northwestern University

It is believed that antibodies might cross the blood-brain barrier and cause damage to certain areas of the brain because of the tau protein shared by brain and sperm. A study by Northwestern University researchers showed an increase in frontotemporal dementia (FTD) in 37% of men who had a vasectomy. FTD is manifested with changes in personality, ability to concentrate, social skills, motivation and reasoning and eventually they develop loss in memory and other brain functions.

The research done at Northwestern University proved that vasectomies may put men at risk for a type of dementia known as Primary Progressive Aphasia (PPA). PPA is a form of dementia that involves a decline in language functions such as speaking.

Epididymitis is one of the most common vasectomy-related complications. This condition occurs when the larger tube behind the testicle, connected to the vas deferens, becomes inflamed and swollen.

Another of the more common abnormal conditions resulting from vasectomy is sperm granulomas. This occurs when sperm leakage from the testicular cut end of the vas deferens causes a benign lump.

Some men develop post-vasectomy pain syndrome, which manifests during intercourse, ejaculation or both. Pain may also come with common physical exertion. The causes of this syndrome are many and may require treatment that could include nerve blockers, pain management, surgical excision of a granuloma and psychiatric referral. In some patients vasectomy reversal is indicated. However, there is a reason why doctors say sterilization by vasectomies is intended to be permanent. Surgery to reverse a vasectomy is complicated and is not always successful.

There are still other concerns:

- hypoglycemia
- diabetes mellitus
- skin eruptions
- itching, hives
- inflamed prostate gland, prostate cancer
- swelling
- bruising
- bleeding
- blood clot in the scrotum
- blood in the semen

- stones in the urinary tract
- thrombophlebitis
- lymph node enlargement
- inflammation
- intense sleepiness
- hormonal imbalance
- infection at the incision site or in deeper tissue
- pain
- depression, anxiety
- erectile dysfunction and/or decreased libido

As if all of this were not enough, there is a small chance that a man who has had a vasectomy may still impregnate a woman. This can occur if the cut vas deferens spontaneously reconnects. In fact, a woman in Seattle, Washington became pregnant even though her husband had undergone a vasectomy. Their doctor discovered that the vas deferens had reconnected so the woman's husband submitted to a second operation. After yet another pregnancy shortly, a third vasectomy was done. In total, this one man had six vasectomy operations. The vas deferens has spontaneously reconnected after every surgery.

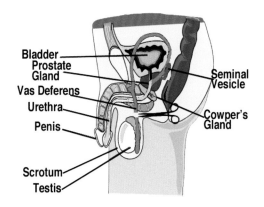

References

Jared M. Baeten, et. al., "Hormonal contraception and risk of sexually transmitted disease acquisition: results from a prospective study", *American Journal of Obstetrics & Gynecology*, August 2001

Neil H. Baum, M.D., et. al, "Vasectomy Risks and Complications" vasectomy.com, circa 2001

Cory G. Christiansen and Jay I. Sandlow, "Testicular Pain Following Vasectomy: A Review of Postvasectomy Pain Syndrome", *Journal of Andrology*, May-June 2003

R. Colović, et.al., "Actinomycosis of the caecum simulating carcinoma in a patient with a long-term intrauterine device", Srpski Arhiv Za Celokupno Lekarstvo (*Serbian Archives for Overall Lekarstvo*), May-June 2009

Robert F. Conkling, "Medicine that makes you sick," January 15, 2010

K.M. Curtis, and S.L. Martins, "Progestogen-only contraception and bone mineral density: a systematic review", *Contraception*, May 2006

Annette B. Ramírez de Arellano, & Conrad Seipp, *Colonialism, Catholicism, and Contraception: A History of Birth Control in Puerto Rico* (Chapel Hill: University of North Carolina Press, 1983)

David Delvin, M.D., "The mini-Pill (progestogen-only Pill, or POP)", NetDoctor, May 31, 2011

Jim Edwards, "Bad Patch", *Brandweek*, August 6, 2007

Yagi Eiichi, et. al, "The ability of four catechol estrogens of 17β-estradiol and estrone to induce DNA adducts in Syrian hamster embryo fibroblasts", *Carcinogenesis* (Oxford University Press, 2001)

Sandra Tarragón Gabarró, et.al, "Accidental introduction of a contraceptive vaginal ring into the urinary bladder", *International Urogynecology Journal and Pelvic Floor Dysfunction*, December 2009

Edward Giovannucci, et.al., "A retrospective cohort study of vasectomy and prostate cancer in US men", *Journal of the American Medical Association*, February 16, 1993

MI Gökce, et.al., "Squamous cell carcinoma of the bladder associated with chronic irritation related to a migrated intrauterine device", *Scandinavian Journal of Urology and Nephrology*, April 2010

David A. Grimes, "Contraceptive implants and injectables: recent developments", *The Contraception Report*, 2000

Daniel T Halperin, et. al., "The time has come for common ground on preventing sexual transmission of HIV", *The Lancet*, November 27, 2004

Robert A. Hatcher, MD, MPH, et. al., *Contraceptive Technology*, 18th ed. (New York: Ardent Media, 2004)

Robert A. Hatcher, M.D., MPH, et. al., *Managing Contraception*, 7th ed. (USA: The Bridging the Gap Foundation, 2004-2005)

W.M. Jordan, & J.K. Anand, "Pulmonary embolism", *The Lancet*, November 18, 1961

Suzanne White Junod & Lara Marks, "Women's Trials: The Approval of the First Oral Contraceptive Pill in the United States and Great Britain", *Journal of the History of Medicine and Allied Sciences*, April 2002

Chris Kahlenborn, M.D., et. al., "Oral Contraceptive Use as a Risk Factor for Premenopausal Breast Cancer: A Meta-analysis", *Mayo Clinic Proceedings*, October 2006

Sefa Kelecia, et.al, "Risk factors for tubal ligation: Regret and psychological effects impact of Beck depression inventory", *Contraception*, June 2005

Cameron D. Klug, et.al., "Fatal toxic shock syndrome from an intrauterine device", *Annals of Emergency Medicine*, November 2009

Richard A. Kronmal, et. al., "Vasectomy and Urolithiasis", *The Lancet*, January 9, 1988

Zehra Kurdoglu, et.al., "Ectopic Intrauterine Device in the Bladder of a Pregnant Woman", *Case Reports in Medicine*, 2010

O.A. Ladipo and S.A. Akinso, "Contraceptive Implants", *African Journal of Reproductive Health*, April 2005

Walter L. Larimore, M.D., "To the Editor", *American Family Physician*, September 1, 1999

L. Luo, et.al., Psychological long-term effects of sterilization on anxiety and depression", *Contraception*, 1996

Albert Q. Maisel, *The Hormone Quest* (New York: Random House, 1965)

Lara V. Marks, *Sexual Chemistry: A History of the Contraceptive Pill* (New Haven: Yale University Press, 2001)

Harold L. Martin, Jr., et. al., "Hormonal contraception, sexually transmitted diseases, and risk of heterosexual transmission of human immunodeficiency virus type 1", *Journal of Infectious Diseases*, October 1998

Charles S. Morrison, Ph.D., et. al., "Hormonal contraception and the risk of HIV acquisition", *AIDS*, January 2, 2007

Charles S. Morrison, Ph.D., et. al., "Hormonal Contraceptive Use, Cervical Ectopy, and the Acquisition of Cervical Infections", *Sexually Transmitted Diseases*, September 2004

Pascal Mourtialon, et. al., "Vascular complication after insertion of a subcutaneous contraceptive implant", *Acta Obstetricia et Gynecologica Scandinavica*, November 2008

Michael Abiola Okunlola, et.al., "Study on Vaginitis Among Intrauterine Contraceptive Device Users in Ibadan, South-western Nigeria", *Journal of Reproduction and Contraception*, December 2009

Ralf G. Rahwan, *Chemical Contraceptives, Interceptives and Abortifacients* (Columbus, Ohio: Ohio State University College of Pharmacy, Division of Pharmacology, 1995)

James Reed, From Private Vice to Public Virtue: *The Birth Control Movement and American Society Since 1830* (New York: Basic Books, 1978)

Edris Rice-Wray, "Field Study with Enovid as a Contraceptive Agent", *Proceedings of a Symposium on 19-Nor Progestational Steroids* (Chicago: Searle Research Laboratories, 1957)

H.J. Roberts, *Is Vasectomy Safe?* (West Palm Beach, Florida: Sunshine Academic Press, 1979)

Bob Roehr, "Hormonal Contraceptives Increase HIV Risk and Disease Progression", *Medscape Medical News*, Report on the 10th Conference on Retroviruses and Opportunistic Infections: Abstract 116, February 12, 2003

Jeff Rosen and Robert Powell, "Did Drugmaker Hide Birth Control Patch Risks", MSNBC News, September 22, 2010

Michael H. Ross, et.al., *Histología. Texto y Atlas color con Biología Celular y Molecular (Histology: Text and Color Atlas and Molecular Cell Biology),* 5th edition, (Mexico: Panamericana, 2007)

Rita Rubin, "Contraceptive is linked to high STD risk", *USA Today*, August 22, 2004

M.J. Sparrow, "Pregnancies in reliable pill takers," *New Zealand Medical Journal*, November 8, 1989

Joseph A. Spinnato II, M.D., "Mechanism of action of intrauterine contraceptive devices and its relation to informed consent", *American Journal of Obstetrics & Gynecology*, March 1997

Joseph B. Stanford, M.D., MSPH, and Rafael T. Mikolajczyk, M.D., "Mechanisms of action of intrauterine devices: Update and estimation of postfertilization effects", *American Journal of Obstetrics & Gynecology (AJOG Reviews)*, December 2002

Lily J. Tythan, "Ortho-Tri Cyclen Lo Side Effects," November 27, 2009 (livestrong.com/article/40600-orthotri-cyclen-lo-side-effects)

Nine Van der Vange, M.D., State University of Utrecht, Department of Obstetrics & Gynecology, *Second International Conference of the Society for Advancement in Contraception, Jakarta, Indonesia,* November 26-30,1984

J.N. Wasserheit, "Epidemiologic synergy: Interrelationships between human immunodeficiency virus infection and other sexually transmitted diseases", *Sexually Transmitted Diseases*, March-April 1992

Sandra Weintraub, et.al, "Vasectomy in men with Primary Progressive Aphasia", *Cognitive & Behavioral Neurology*, December 2006

Sandra Weintraub, "Vasectomy May Put Men at Risk for Type of Dementia," Cognitive Neurology and Alzheimer's Disease Center, Northwestern University Feinberg School of Medicine, *Annual Report 2007*, February 13, 2007

E. Weisberg, "Oral Contraceptives: Fine Tuning Clinical Use," *Patient Management*, July 1988

John Wilks, B.Pharm. M.S., *A Consumer's Guide to The Pill and Other Drugs*, 2nd ed. (Stafford, Virg.: ALL Inc., 1997)

John Wilks, B. Pharm, M.S., M.A.C., "The Pill: How It Works and Fails" (Stafford, Virg.: ALL Inc., 2002)

I.C. Winter, "Industrial pressure and the population problem–the FDA and the pill", *Journal of the American Medical Association*, May 1970

"The Role of STD Prevention and Treatment in HIV Prevention", *CDC Fact Sheet*, December 2007 (updated September 2010)

"The Single-Rod Contraceptive Implant", *Clinical Proceedings, Association of Reproductive Health Professionals*, July 2008

"Post Tubal Syndrome (PTS) Symptom List", The Coalition for Post Tubal Ligation Women

"Dear Healthcare Organization Leader", letter from Pfizer Inc., November 18, 2004

"Dear Healthcare Professional", letter from Pfizer Inc., November 18, 2004

Depo-Provera CI, "Full Prescribing Information", Pfizer Inc. (Pharmacia & Upjohn Company), July 2011

"Black Box Warning Added Concerning Long-Term Use of Depo-Provera Contraceptive Injection", Doc Guide, Doctor's Guide Publishing Ltd., 2005

"Implanon contraceptive implant: changing to Nexplanon", Medicines and Healthcare products Regulatory Agency (MHRA), "Drug Safety Update", October 2010 (revised January 14, 2011)

"Hormonal contraception and bone health", *Family Planning, World Health Organization*, September 5, 2005

"Oral Contraceptives: Requirement for Labeling Directed to the Patient", U.S. Food and Drug Administration, Department of Health, Education and Welfare, *Federal Register*, January 31, 1978

"Statement of Policy Concerning Oral Contraceptive Labeling Directed to Users", U.S. Food and Drug Administration, *Federal Register*, June 11, 1970

"Oral Contraceptives: Patient Package Insert Requirement", U.S. Food and Drug Administration, *Federal Register*, May 25, 1989

"Black Box Warning Added Concerning Long-Term Use of Depo-Provera Contraceptive Injection", Find Law, Thomson Reuters Corporation, November 2004

"Los anticonceptivos hormonales pueden afectar a la feminidad" ("Hormonal contraceptives may affect femininity"), Forum Libertas, November 28, 2008

"Progestin-only Contraceptives", Hall Health Primary Care Center, University of Washington, September 13, 2010

"Implanon (etonogestrel implant)", U.S. product information, N.V. Organon (subsidiary of Merck & Company), 2006 (rev. March 2009)

"Ectopic Pregnancy", Kids Health, The Nemours Foundation, February 2008

Mirena (levonorgestrel-releasing intrauterine system), U.S. product information, Bayer HealthCare Pharmaceuticals Inc., 2009

"Update: Barrier Protection Against HIV Infection and Other Sexually Transmitted Diseases", *MMWR (Morbidity and Mortality Weekly Report)*, Centers for Disease Control and Prevention, August 6, 1993

"Vasectomy may put men at risk for dementia", Northwestern University, February 12, 2007; updated January 9, 2010

"NuvaRing (etonogestrel/ethinyl estradiol vaginal ring)", U.S. product information, N.V. Organon (subsidiary of Merck & Company), 2008

"ACOG Committee Opinion No, 415: Depot medroxyprogesterone

acetate and bone effects", American College of *Obstetricians and Gynecologists*, Committee on Gynecologic Practice, Obstetrics and Gynecology, September 2008

"Ortho Evra Transdermal System", *Ortho Women's Health & Urology*, May 2005

Ortho Tri-Cyclen Lo Tablets (norgestimate/ethinyl estradiol)", U.S. product information, Janssen Pharmaceuticals (subsidiary of Johnson & Johnson) Inc., 1998 (rev. 2010)

ParaGard (intrauterne copper contraceptive), U.S. product information, "Duramed Pharmaceuticals (subsidiary of Teva Pharmaceutical Industries Ltd.), 2006

"Exposure to DMPA in pregnancy may cause low birth weight", *Progress in Human Reproduction Research*, 1992

"Pathology Picture of the Month", *Surgical Rounds*, December 1980

"Black Box Warning Added Concerning Long-Term Use of Depo-Provera Contraceptive Injection", U.S. Food and Drug Administration, November 17, 2004

"Carcinogenicity of combined hormonal contraceptives and combined menopausal treatment", UNDP/UNFPA/WHO/World Bank Special Programme of Research-Development and Research Training in Human Reproduction (HRP), September 2005

"A Warning on Depo-Provera, *The Washington Post*, November 18, 2004

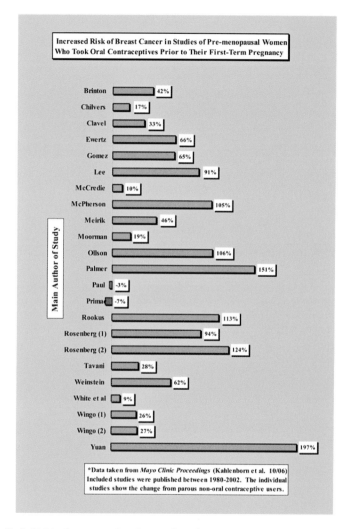

Dr. Chris Kahlenborn practices Internal Medicine in Camp Hill, PA and is the current President of the Polycarp Research Institute (www.polycarp.org). He is the author of Breast Cancer, Its Link to Abortion and the Birth Control Pill.

Breast Cancer Risk from The Pill

By Chris Kahlenborn, MD

Two of the most important types of hormones that control reproduction are estrogens and progestins. Birth control pills are made from synthetic estrogens and/or progestins. Experiments have shown that these hormones cause women's breast cells to divide more rapidly. [1] Cells which divide more rapidly are more prone to develop into cancer cells.

In 2005, the World Health Organization classified oral contraceptives as a Group I carcinogen—the most dangerous classification known.[2] Also, a comprehensive meta-analysis published in the Mayo Clinic Proceedings in October, 2006[3] found that 21 out of 23 retrospective studies done since 1980 showed that women who took oral contraceptive prior to the birth of their first child sustained a 44% average increased risk of developing pre-menopausal breast cancer, [see Table p. 159] "This risk rose to 52% for women who took the pill for at least four years prior to the birth of their first child."

Breast cancer is the most common cause of cancer death in U. S. in women age 20-59. In the U.S. about 211,000 women are diagnosed annually and over 40,000 die from this disease.[4] More than one in five women who are diagnosed with breast cancer (ie, 47,000 women annually) will develop it before menopause. About one in eight women will develop breast cancer at some time in her life and one fourth of such women will die from this disease. Using the birth control pill, especially at a young age, markedly increases a woman's risk for developing breast cancer. This risk is increased even higher when combined with other breast cancer risk factors such as induced abortion, hormone treatment (such as estrogen supplementation), family history of breast cancer, and other factors.

Research studies show that breast cancer risk is almost tripled for women who used Depo-Provera for 2 years or more before age 25. [5]

Oral contraceptives decrease the risk of ovarian and uterine cancer, while they increase the risk of cervical and breast cancer. [6] Since breast cancer is far more prevalent than the other three types of gynecological cancers, the pills overall effect is detrimental to women.

Well known side effects of the Pill include an increased frequency of blood clots, high blood pressure, and heart attacks, as well as migraines, depression, loss of libido, and a variety of other disorders. Less well known is that oral contraceptives and injectable progestins (such as *Depo-Provera*) significantly increase the risk of contracting and transmitting HIV (the AIDS virus). [7,8] In addition, medical studies strongly suggest that oral contraceptives work at times by causing an early abortion. [9]

Many of the known risk factors for breast cancer can be avoided: hormone exposure (including hormonal contraceptives), induced abortion, heavy alcohol use, obesity, and radiation exposure. In addition, there is a significant reduction of risk with each child a woman bears. Every month of breastfeeding reduces breast cancer risk, as does bearing a child at a younger age. Some medications (e.g., raloxifene) which are taken after menopause to help strengthen bones have been shown to markedly reduce the risk of postmenopausal breast cancer and should be considered by all women at high risk.[10]

Natural Family Planning (NFP) methods are available which use no chemicals or surgery and cause no increase in breast cancer risk. Not to be confused with the rhythm method, NFP is based on observations of a woman's cervical mucus and (for some methods) other symptoms as well. One of the largest research studies of NFP (involving 19,843 women and performed in India by the World Health Organization) showed a pregnancy rate of 0.2 pregnancies per 100 women yearly. [11]

Natural Family Planning methods have been used to diagnose and treat a variety of female reproductive disorders including infertility. Various medical problems (e.g., excessive menstrual cramping and bleeding), which are sometimes treated with contraceptive hormones, can be treated far more safely with less toxic means (e.g., magnesium/calcium supplements and/or ibuprofen products).

Anyone may download the Mayo Clinic meta-analysis article by going to www.MayoClinicProceedings.com. In addition, eleven of the seventeen chapters in the book Breast Cancer, Its Link to Abortion and the Birth Control Pill deal with cancer risks from birth control pills. [6]

References

1. Anderson T, Battersby S, et al. Oral contraceptive use influences resting breast proliferation. Hum. Pathol. 1989; 20: 1139-1144.

2. World Health Organization International Agency for Research on Cancer. IARC Monographs. July 29, 2005.

3. Kahlenborn C, Modugno FM et al. Oral contraceptive use as a risk factor for premenopausal breast cancer: a meta-analysis. Mayo Clin Proc. 2006;81(10):1290-1302.

4. Breast Cancer Facts and Figures 2003-2004. American Cancer Society. (www.cancer.org)

5. Skegg DCG, Noonan EA, et al. Depot medroxyprogesterone acetate and breast cancer [A pooled analysis of the World Health Organization and New Zealand studies]. JAMA. 1995;799-804.

6. Kahlenborn C. Breast Cancer, Its Link to Abortion and the Birth Control Pill. One More Soul, Dayton, 2000.

7. Ungchusak, et al. Determinants of HIV infection among female commercial sex workers in northern Thailand: results from a longitudinal study. J Ac Immune Defic Syn Hum Retro. 1996. 12: 500-507.

8. Mostad SB, et al. Hormonal contraception, vitamin A deficiency and other risk factors for shedding HIV-1 infected cells from the cervix and the vagina. The Lancet 1997. 350: 922-927

9. Larimore WL, Stanford J. Postfertilization effects of oral contraceptives and their relationship to informed consent. Arch Fam Med. 9; 2000: 126-133

10. National Cancer Institute. Study of tamoxifen and raloxifene (STAR) trial. April 26, 2006. (www.cancer.gov/star)

11. Ryder RE. Natural Family Planning: Effective birth control supported by the Catholic Church. Br Med J. 1993; 307: 723-726.

XI.

Normal Breast Physiology and Breast Cancer Risk

There are 4 types of lobules whose structural differences appear under the microscope

- These lobules represent different stages of development and maturity of breast tissue.
- Type 1, 2 and 3 lobules are differentiatd by the *average number of ductules per lobular unit*.
- Type 1 has *11*; Type 2 has *47*; Type 3 has *80*.
- Type 4 lobules are fully matured and contain colostrum or milk.

Structural differences that appear under the microscope

- Type 1 lobules mature into Type 2 lobules under the cyclic influence of the female hormones, estrogen and progesterone, during menstrual cycles.
- Type 2 lobules only become fully mature into Type 3 then Type 4 lobules under the influence of the hormonal changes of a full-term pregnancy.

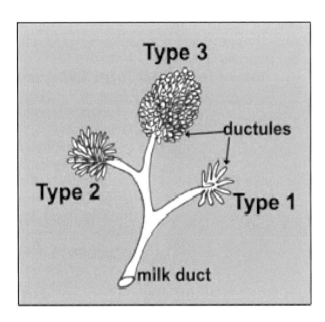

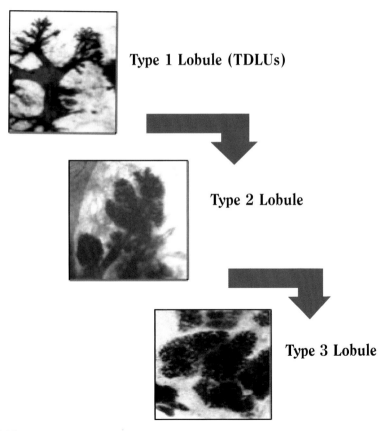

Type 1 Lobule (TDLUs)

Type 2 Lobule

Type 3 Lobule

Hormonal influences for breast lobule development

- A major influence in this final stage of maturation into Type 4 lobules is human placental lactogen (hPL), which sharply rises during the second half of pregnancy.
- Human chorionic gonadotropin (hCG), which stimulates the ovaries to produce estrogen and progesterone within a few days after conception and prolactin, also play a major role in maturation.
- hCG and hPL are made in the mother's womb during pregnancy.

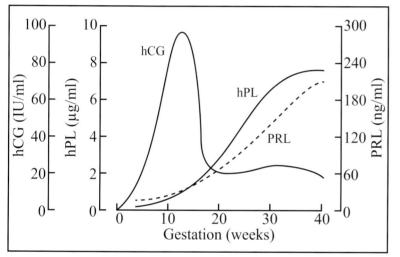

- hPL made by the fetal-placental unit during pregnancy induces full differentiation of breast tissue to Type 4 lobules, which are cancer resistant.
- When Type 4 lobules regress to Type 3 post-weaning, Type 3 lobules are cancer resistant.
- hCG also stimulates the ovary to produce inhibin, a cancer suppressing hormone, increasing protection of the mother even more.

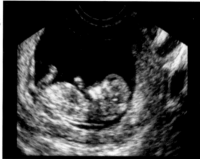

What is the link between estrogen and breast cancer?

Estrogen can cause cancer in two ways:

- As promoter: Estrogen promotes breast tissue to a fast increase in the number of cells. This may result in cancer due to errors in copying the DNA (genes).

  - Type 1 and 2 lobules have more estrogen and progesterone receptors than Type 3.
  - They grow through mitosis (cell division) when estrogen and progesterone levels are elevated.

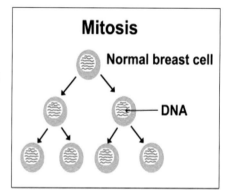

165

- As carcinogen: Certain metabolites of estrogen directly damage DNA, thereby causing cancer cells to form.

  - Mitosis requires replication of DNA and, therefore, can result in mutations.
  - This growth (proliferation) under estrogen and progesterone stimulation explains the cancer causing properties of estrogen/progestin combination drugs (all hormonal methods).

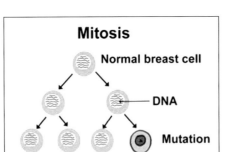

These 4 types of lobules are also metabolically different with different breast cancer potential

- Mutated cells also undergo mitosis.
- Multiple mutations can cause cancer cells to form.
- Cells of Type 1 and 2 lobules also multiply faster than Type 3 resulting in more chances for mutations to occur.
- This growth (proliferation) under estrogen and progesterone stimulation explains the cancer causing properties of estrogen/progestin combination drugs.

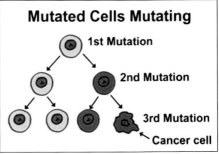

It often takes many repeated exposures to carcinogens before the DNA sustains enough damage that a cancer cell is formed. Although a person may form cancer cells many times during life, the body's immune system can keep these cells from reproducing, and destroys them. It is only when a large number of cancer cells have reproduced that we can be aware of these cells (on average it takes 8-10 years before one breast cancer cell multiplies enough times to cause a cancerous tumor ½ inch in diameter to form).

The risk factors of estrogen exposure and breast immaturity can also act in concert with one another, causing greater risk. For example, if a teenager, who has not had a full-term pregnancy (she is nulliparous), takes birth control pills, her risk of breast cancer is much higher because she was exposed to the carcinogen and promoter effects of estrogen when her lobules were more susceptible to cancer. (See Lobular Structures in the Human Breast on page 164.)

The breast maturation process through a normal full-term pregnancy

At birth:

- After the mother's hormones dissipate, a small amount of breast tissue lies dormant under the infant's nipple and areola.

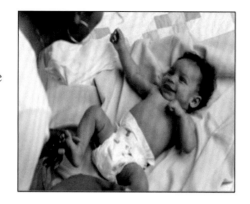

At puberty:

- When the ovaries produce cyclic elevations of the female sex steroid hormones, estrogen and progesterone, the breast enlarges.
- However, only Type 1 and 2 lobules are formed, which are where ductal and lobular cancers start respectively.
- Most of the breast tissue is stroma (tissue surrounding the lobules).
- The lobules account for about 10% of the breast tissue.

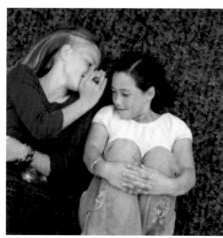

After puberty:

- There is a reduction in stroma and lobules now account for 30% of the breast tissue.
- The breast is now:

  - 75% Type 1
  - 25% Type 2 lobules with a few Type 3

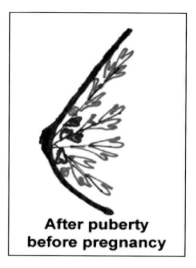

After puberty before pregnancy

After conception:

- The baby secretes human Chorionic Goanadotrophins (hCG)
  - Stimulating the ovaries to produce the pregnancy hormones estrogen and progesterone
  - Causing the breast to start to enlarge by making *greater numbers of lobules*.
  - Causing the mother's breast to feel sore and tender.

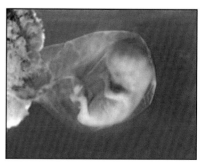

By the end of the 1st trimester:

- During the maturation of Type 1 lobules into Type 2, the actual *numbers of these lobules will increase* while the surrounding tissue (stroma) deceases.
- The breast now has *more places for cancers to start*.

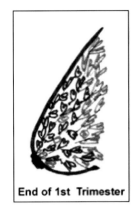

End of 1st Trimester

By the end of the 3rd trimester:

- **The breast is now:**

  - 85% Type 4 lobules.
  - 15% immature cancer susceptible lobules.

There are now *fewer places for cancer to start*.

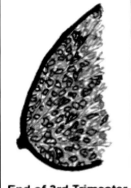

End of 3rd Trimester

By mid 2nd trimester:

- The breast has *doubled in volume* and has continued to mature rapidly under the influence of placental lactogen.
- **The breast is now:**

  - 70% Type 4 cancer resistant lobules.
  - 30% immature cancer susceptible lobules.

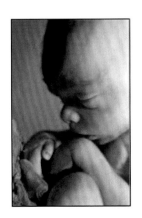

At delivery:

- The mother's breasts are now *predominantly Type 4 lobules*.
- They are fully mature and resistant to carcinogens.
- *There are fewer places for breast cancer to start*.
- This results in lower long-term risk of breast cancer for the mother.

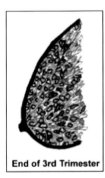

End of 3rd Trimester

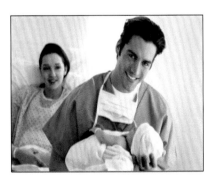

Lobular Structures in the Human Breast

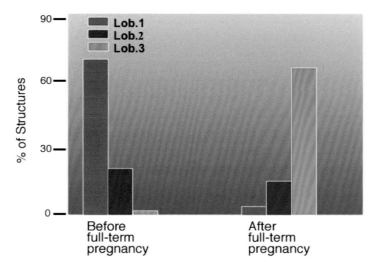

Breast lobule maturation before and after first pregnancy

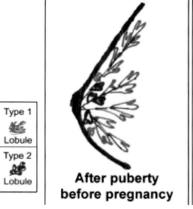

After puberty before pregnancy

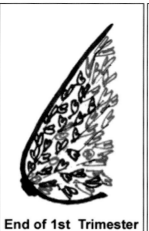

End of 1st Trimester

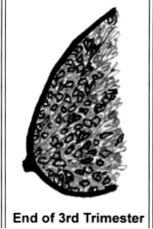

End of 3rd Trimester

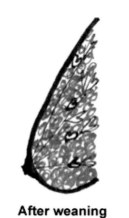

After weaning

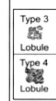

While breastfeeding:

- The breast tissue is maximally differentiated to Type 4 lobules.
- The mother's menstrual cycles may stop or become anovulatory, further reducing her risk.

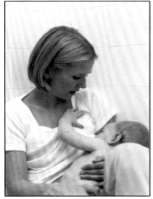

After weaning:

- Type 4 lobules regress to Type 3 and the breasts get smaller again.
- However, there is evidence of *permanent changes in the genes* of these Type 3 lobules which confer *life-long cancer resistance* even after menopause when they further regress to Type 1.

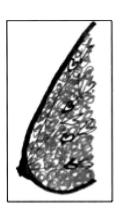
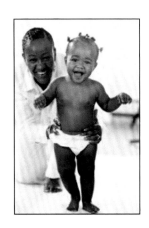

These facts about the breast maturation process account for the following known facts about breast cancer risk:

- A woman who has a full-term pregnancy decreases her breast cancer risk.
- A woman who is childless has increased breast cancer risk.

The "susceptibility window"

- The period between puberty and a full-term pregnancy
- The time the breast is most susceptible to forming cancer, i.e., when the woman's breast is composed primarily of Type 1 and 2 lobules.

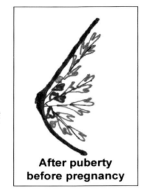

After puberty before pregnancy

How is it that Lobules Type 1 and Type 2 are more susceptible to cancer?

Lobules Type 1 and Type 2 copy their DNA faster than Type 3 lobules. DNA contains all the information of a cell. The faster DNA is copied, the higher the risk of copying wrong information and the new cells are created with changes (mutations) that could lead to cancer.

- *If* a woman does not have a full-term pregnancy (meaning she is childless or nulliparous), she has increased risk for breast cancer, since she never developed Type 4 lobules.
- *If* she had children later in life (after age 30), she has increased risk, because for most of her menstrual life, her estrogen has been stimulating immature Type 1 and 2 breast lobules.

What is the link between abortion and breast cancer?

A woman who gets pregnant increases her estrogen level 2,000% by the end of the first trimester. If it ends before 32 weeks (by very premature birth or induced abortion), she was exposed to estrogen without having the benefit of full breast maturation; she has more places for breast cancer to start. Spontaneous abortions (miscarriages) in the first trimester do not increase breast cancer risk because they are associated with low estrogen levels.

Types of Breast Lobules

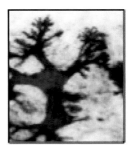

Type 1 Lobule (TDLUs)

95% of all breast cancers arise in Type 1 Lobules (Ductal cancer)

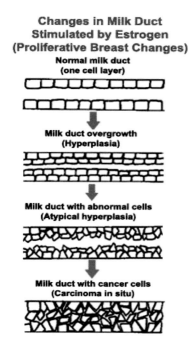

Estrogen promotes a fast increase in the number of cells, which may result in errors while copying DNA

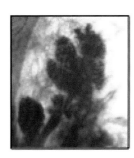

Type 2 Lobule

10% of all breast cancers arise in Type 2 Lobules (Lobular cancer)

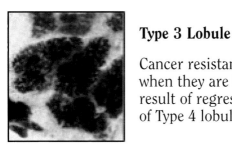

Type 3 Lobule

Cancer resistant when they are the result of regression of Type 4 lobules

Source: Lanfranchi, Angela and Brind, Joel; <u>Breast Cancer: Risk and Prevention,</u> 4th ed. available at: www.bcpinstitute.org/booklet4.htm.

ADDITIONAL STUDIES

Study funded by the National Institute of Cancer in woman under 45 years of age that had one or more induced abortions

Researchers from the Fred Hutchinson Cancer Center of Seattle, Washington, discovered that women who had been pregnant at least once, and those who had an induced abortion, had a 50% higher risk of contracting breast cancer than those who had never had abortions. The risk was higher among those who had abortions before age 18 or after 30 years of age. Between those two groups, the risk of breast cancer increases if abortion took place between the 8th and 12th week of pregnancy. This study confirmed the theory that the link between the risk of breast cancer and induced abortion is due to the differentiation of the structures of the lobules of the mammary gland. The mammary gland appears to be the only organ that is not fully developed at birth. It changes dramatically in size, form and function in response to growth, puberty, pregnancy and breast feeding.

What happens if there is breast cancer in my family?

Women who have a history of breast cancer in their family and decide to have an induced abortion have a very high risk of developing breast cancer. Women with a history of breast cancer in their family who have had two or more induced abortions had a 600% increased risk factor of developing breast cancer, compared to the rest of the population. Daling, et al. 1994 observed that women who had an abortion before age 18 and had a family history of breast cancer had an infinitely higher risk of developing breast cancer compared with young women who had a history of breast cancer in the family but did not have induced abortions. She also observed that women who were 30 years or older when they had induced abortions and had a history of breast cancer in their family, had an increased risk of 270%.

But isn't pregnancy and birth more dangerous than abortion?

No. The risk of breast cancer increases with induced abortion. The risk of suicide is far higher after an abortion, however, the risk of ovarian cancer is reduced after the pregnancy comes to term.

If a woman develops breast cancer during pregnancy, should she abort the baby?

Definitely not. A woman diagnosed with breast cancer while pregnant has a higher probability of living longer if she gives birth than if she aborts. In 1989, Clark and Chase found in their study that women who had breast cancer did not survive past 5 years after having an abortion, while 20% of women that had breast cancer who chose to give birth were alive after 11 years.

Additional Studies

Study financed by the National Cancer Institute (Fred Hutchinson Center of Cancer Research and the Department of Epidemiology of the University of Washington in Seattle).

Results of Study of Risks of Breast Cancer due to induced Abortion (before age 45).

Regarding Ages 18 - 30: Although highest risks are observed when abortion is done at ages younger than 18 (particularly if it occurs after 8 weeks gestation) or at age 30 or older, data in NCI funded study supports the hypothesis that an induced abortion at any age can advsersely influence a woman's subsequent risk of breast cancer.

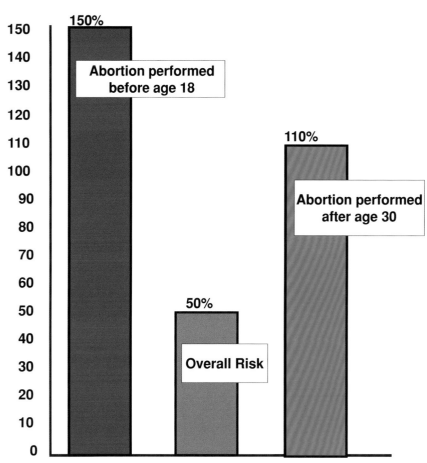

SOURCE: Journal of the National Cancer Institute. 86 No. 21 (November 2, 1994).
The Houston Chronicles. October 26,1994. P. 10A. By Tom Paulson. Seattle Post-Intelligence.

References:

1. Brind J, Chinchilli M, et al. Induced Abortion as an Independent Risk Factor for Breast Cancer: a Comprehensive review and metaanalisis. J Epidemiol Community Health. 10/1996; 50: 481-496.

2. Landis SH et al. Cancer Statistics. CA Cancer J Clin. 1999; 49: 12-23.

3. Daling J, Malone K, et al. Risk of Breast Cancer Among Young Women: Relationship to Induce Abortion. JNCI. 1994; 86: 1584-1592.

4. Andrieu N, et al. Familial Risk of Breast Cancer and Abortion. Cancer Detection and Prevention. 1994; 18: 51-55.

5. Ryder RE. "Natural Family Planning." Effective Birth Control Supported by the Catholic Church. Br Med J. 1993; 307: 723-726.

6. Clarck RM, Chua T. Breast Cancer and Pregnancy: The Ultimate Challenge. Clinical Oncology. 1989; 1: 11-18.

Article published in: One More Soul. Dayton, Ohio. United States. 2009 Available at: www.oms.com.

Doctor Chris Kahlenborn is an internal medicine physician who practices in Altoona, Pa. Doctor Kahlenborn is the author of the book: Breast Cancer, Its Link to Abortion and the Birth Control Pill. One More Soul USA/Canada. 2000.

XII.

ATTENTION PREGNANT MOTHERS

Cord Blood:
Who Owns It?

Cord Blood -- Who Owns It?

By Mercedes Arzú Wilson and Paul A. Byrne, M.D.

INTRODUCTION

The purpose of providing this important knowledge is to remind the parents that the umbilical cord blood, first and foremost, belongs to the baby; not only before birth but also immediately after birth. The baby is NOT to be depleted of these basic nutrients that are needed for circulation to the lungs after birth.

The parents or researchers will be able to preserve what is left ONLY after the baby has taken what he or she needs. Cord blood banks are expanding without factual information as to the true merits of this new research. Hence, many couples are falling prey of an emerging multi-million dollar business.

Life on Earth is a continuum from conception until true death.

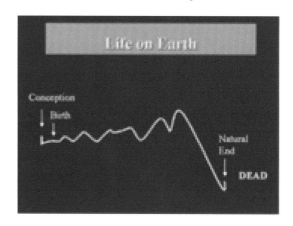

The life of a human person is manifested at the moment of conception, when the invisible becomes visible, creating an explosion of life as the soul enters the body. At that moment, the child receives his genetic make-up. Twenty-three chromosomes from his mother and twenty-three chromosomes from his father.

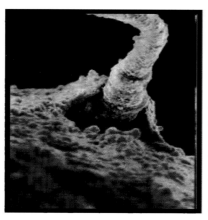

The early life of the baby is spent within his private intrauterine environment, the amniotic fluid, which is made wholly and entirely by the infant himself.

Life on earth after birth depends on whatever happens before and during birth. Large volumes of blood in the umbilical cord and placenta are needed for the volume of blood necessary for the increased blood flow to the baby's lungs after birth.

We are expressing and emphasizing that large volumes of blood are in the umbilical cord and placenta required for circulation immediately after birth, especially to the lungs. Umbilical cord blood belongs to the baby and ought not to be stolen by those who wish to use the umbilical cord blood for experimentation.

The Lungs Before Birth

The lungs before birth are organs of secretion. The movements of the chest push the lung fluid into the amniotic fluid. At birth the lungs must

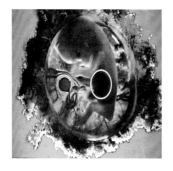 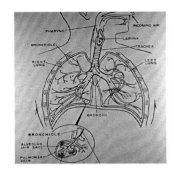

stop producing fluid so they can become an organ of absorption; then air enters the lungs for them to become the organ of respiration.

When does Pulmonary resistance decrease and Pulmonary blood flow increase?

The volume of blood needed for this increased pulmonary flow comes from the blood in the umbilical cord, unless the doctors mistakenly clamp the cord immediately too close to the "navel" in order to get blood

Clamping of the Cord

Early	vs.	Late
1. Facilitates resuscitation		1. Oxygen until placenta separation
2. Treatment of mother		2. Transfusion to infant (60-200 ml. Blood)

Position of Infant
Stripping of Cord
Length of Cord

to save for stem cells. When the cord has been clamped immediately and short, the circulation very likely is "robbed" from the baby.

This drawing shows the narrow terminal bronchioles and the wider alveoli, which before birth are full of fluid. When air replaces this fluid, pressure on the pulmonary capillaries is reduced. This allows increased circulation to the lungs. The volume of blood needed for this increased circulation naturally comes from the umbilical cord blood unless someone disturbs this natural process by clamping the cord quickly and close to the newborn infant. Therefore, when the umbilical cord is clamped quickly and close to the infant, the physician robs the infant of the blood necessary for the increased flow to the infant's lungs. To compensate for this the infant must use blood that would otherwise go to the brain, heart, liver, and kidneys. For this powerful reason, it is wrong to clamp the cord quickly and short in order to obtain a large quantity of blood to use for stem cell research, experimentation, and possible use later by the infant and others.

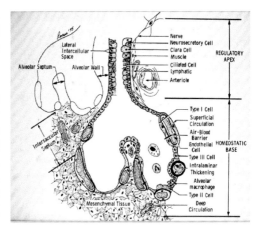

Delayed clamping of the cord or clamping it as far away from the baby as possible allows a natural transfusion of 60 to 200 mL of blood into the infant. This is equivalent to 1 to 2 transfusion units of blood for an adult.

It is imperative that the parents recognize that the umbilical cord blood belongs to the baby. The baby's parents must be properly informed so that they can responsibly protect and preserve the life of their baby given to them by God.

It is essential that a dynamic thought process is in effect when treating and caring for an infant. Information before birth must be obtained and evaluated. The results of fetal monitoring are particularly important especially if there are repeated occurrences of an abnormal fetal heart rate. The presence of meconium in the amniotic fluid, especially in the asphyxiated infant, requires that immediately after birth the mouth be suctioned first and then the nose, here again, leaving the infant with a long cord and allowing time for the blood to go into the baby is essential. The cord must not be milked into the baby or toward the placenta. The infant is evaluated at birth, including Apgar scores. No one should consider taking blood for stem cells until the baby has completely adapted to extrauterine respiration and circulation.

The photograph shows a happy pink baby who would say, "As I enter my new world, thank you for leaving my cord long and allowing me to have my blood that is needed to fill my lungs to prevent respiratory distress, persistent fetal circulation, cerebral hypoxia, intraventricular hemorrhage, anemia, and possibly autism."

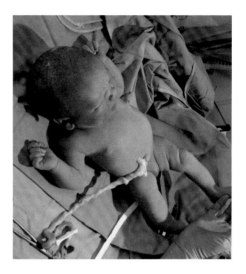

Bibliography

ACOG Committee on Obstetric Practice. ACOG Committee Opinion No 348, November 2006: Umbilical cord blood gas and acid-base analysis. *Obstet Gynecol*. 2006 Nov; 108 (5) :1319-22.

Baenziger O, Stolkin F, Keel M, von Siebenthal K, Fauchere JC, Das Kundu S, Dietz V, Bucher HU, Wolf M. The influence of the timing of cord clamping on postnatal cerebral oxygenation in preterm neonates: a randomized, controlled trial. *Pediatrics*. 2007 Mar;119(3):455-9.

Chaparro CM, Neufeld LM, Tena Alavez G, Eguia-Líz Cedillo R, Dewey KG. Effect of timing of umbilical cord clamping on iron status in Mexican infants: a randomized controlled trial. *Lancet*. 2006 Jun 17; 367 (9527) :1997-2004.

Hutton EK, Hassan ES. Late vs early clamping of the umbilical cord in full-term neonates: systematic review and meta-analysis of controlled trials. *JAMA*. 2007 Mar 21; 297 (11) :1241-52.

Mercer JS, Vohr BR, McGrath MM, Padbury JF, Wallach M, Oh W. Delayed cord clamping in very preterm infants reduces the incidence of intraventricular hemorrhage and late-onset sepsis: a randomized, controlled trial. *Pediatrics*. 2006 Apr; 117 (4) :1235-42.

Mercer JS, McGrath MM, Hensman A, Silver H, Oh W. Immediate and delayed cord clamping in infants born between 24 and 32 weeks: a pilot randomized controlled trial. *J Perinatol*. 2003 Sep; 23 (6) :466-72.

Morley GM. Cord closure: can hasty clamping injure the newborn? *OBG Management*. 1998 Jul; 7:29-36

Oh W. Timing of umbilical cord clamping at birth in full-term infants. *JAMA*. 2007 Mar 21; 297 (11) :1257-8.

Rabe H, Reynolds G, Diaz-Rossello J. Early versus delayed umbilical cord clamping in preterm infants. *Cochrane Database Syst Rev*. 2004 Oct 18;(4):CD003248.

APPENDICES

Who is Family of the Americas?

Family of the Americas Foundation (FAF) is a non-profit organization incorporated in 1977 with its international headquarters in Maryland and branch offices in many parts of the world.

FAF's purpose is to promote family unity by encouraging parents to meet their mutual responsibilities to each other and to their children.

FAF programs include:

1. Natural Family Planning teacher-training programs in over 100 countries, in North America, Europe, Africa, Latin America and Asia, including the People's Republic of China.

2. Development, publication and distribution of educational materials in English, Spanish, French, Italian, German, Hungarian, Czech, Slovak, Korean, Japanese, Chinese, Portuguese, Catalan, Arabic, Swahili, Russian, Lithuanian, Ukrainian, Romanian, and Polish.

3. Clinical and research studies to further scientific knowledge of the Ovulation Method of Natural Family Planning.

4. Programs for parents to encourage them to remain the primary educators of their children in matters of human sexuality.

5. International Congresses for the Family which raise awareness about issues affecting the family.

6. Educational programs in nutrition, hygiene, Oral Rehydration Therapy (ORT) and Natural Family Planning for participants in Latin America.

7. Manufacture water filters for the poor, in order to provide potable water for them.

Profits from the sale of our materials help us to provide these programs and materials to developing countries.

U.S.A.

Master Training class held -- Green Bay, Wisconsin 2011.

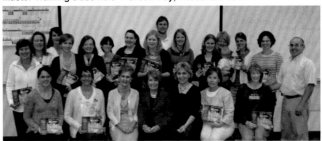

Europe

Over 20 Congresses for the Family, in 16 different countries have been organized by Family of the Americas, this one was held in Vienna, Austria.

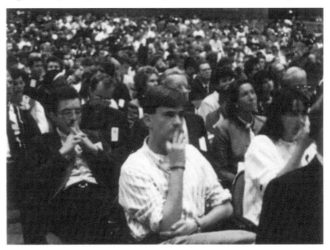

China

Dr. Zhang De-Wei, Deputy Director of Shanghai Municipal Commission of Family Planning, instructs teachers in Shanghai.

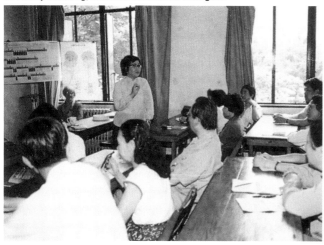

Africa

Representatives from African countries who were trained in the U.S. to teach the Ovulation Method in Africa.

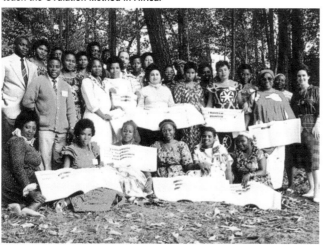

India

Representatives from India and other Asian countries who came to the U.S. to be trained by FAF to teach the Ovulation Method.

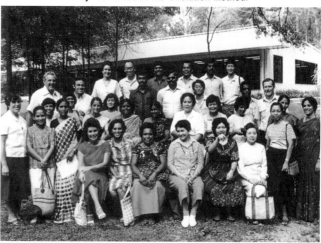

Central America

Instructors in Guatemala teach the Ovulation Method using illustrated posters.

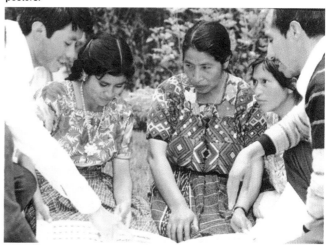

Endorsements of The Method:

Alice von Hildebrand, Ph.D.
Professor Emeritus of Hunter College

Years ago, I was interviewed by an anchor in Portland, OR. Rightly suspecting me to reject materialism, he asked me the following question: "Could you name one essential difference between man and animals"? Without a moment's hesitation, I answered, "Yes, the sexual sphere". The man practically fell off his seat. And yet, one of the many "paradoxes" of Christianity is that things which seem to be similar, or even identical, can, upon a closer look, be at antipodes. It is true indeed that spiritual beings (God and Angels) have no gender. They transcend it, whereas both animals and human beings are divided between "the male and the female" sex. This is a striking similarity. But a closer look reveals that this similarity conceals a radical difference. Whereas the animal male is exclusively attracted to the female when the latter is in heat, this does not apply to human beings. Husband and wife desire "union" at all times, including the days when the wife is infertile. The "intention unionis" is an essential feature of love.

God is the author of nature, and we, His creatures, must learn to read its message. How are we to interpret the striking dissimilarity just mentioned? Alas, our minds being affected by original sin, we are "talented" in misinterpreting the messages God sends us through His creation. Some will read it to mean that man can divorce the unitive and the procreative dimension of the marital embrace, and therefore legitimize artificial birth control in all its forms. In other words, the Devil que nunca duerme, (that never sleeps), tries to hijack this basic difference between men and animals, and uses it to convince them that they are therefore morally justified in willingly separating the two

dimensions. In fact, the book of nature created by God, while acknowledging that the desire for union is an essential characteristic of love, does not entitle us to intentionally separate the "becoming one flesh" from fruitfulness. By its very nature, love is and should be fruitful. But when God Himself closes the levies, the spouses are thereby permitted to experience the sweetness of union when procreation is excluded. But what is severely against God's law and therefore prohibited by the Holy Church, the porta voce of the Creator in matters of faith and morals, is to willingly sever the profound bond existing between the unitive and the procreative dimension. This is the message that NFP shares with us, and its message should be gratefully accepted. Mercedes Wilsons' book sheds abundant light on this fact. NFP is a proof that science is not antagonistic to faith, but must be understood in the light of faith. This book is a must read for all those concerned about this very important problem.

The Late Prof. Jerome Lejeune
Doctor of Medicine and Natural Sciences
Professor of Genetics, The Faculty of Medicine, Paris, France
Director of Research and Fundamental Genetics, The Faculty of Medicine, Paris, France
Chief of the Department of Fundamental Genetics, Pediatric Hospital, Paris, France
Member, Royal College of Medicine
Member, Pontifical Academy of Sciences, Rome
Founder of Pontifical Academy of Life

The perfect scientific procedure of mastering nature is the obedience to its laws. And science reveals to us that the natural regulation of births, or rather of conception, is not only possible but fully effective.

Being able to control the fertility of love without abortion, without an IUD, without a pill and with no artificial method of any kind, is completely contrary to current propaganda. But each woman can determine for herself if her physiological condition will or will not permit her to procreate at a given time. In reality, this basic principle has been known since time immemorial - what farmer would take his mare to stud without having

made sure that she is really in heat? Certainly, the female organism is much more delicately regulated than that of an animal; the signs of fertility at ovulation time are much less obvious. But with the help of feminine intuition, just as she can distinguish by touch between a silk scarf and a square of rayon or between a cotton cloth and synthetic fiber, any woman can recognize the signs of her fertility by learning what to look for.

The awareness of fertility is the basis for the true freedom of love.

The Late Walker Percy, M.D.
Fellow of the American Academy of Arts & Sciences
Member of the National Institute of Arts & Sciences
Recipient of the National Book Award '62

This is a very useful manual on the Billings Ovulation Method, which is a practical method of family planning for those couples who wish to have a child or to avoid having a child—and to do so without using mechanical methods of contraception or introducing chemicals into their bodies.

What makes this book particularly useful is that it combines Mercedes Wilson's very clear explanation of the way a woman's body works, which any high school student can understand—this, with a sophisticated appendix explaining the physiology and endocrinology of the menstrual cycle.

Arman M. Nicholi, Jr., M.D.
Associate Clinical Professor of Psychiatry, Harvard Medical School

Mercedes Wilson has written an excellent book that clearly describes a natural method for family planning. Love and Fertility beautifully illustrates the Ovulation Method for determining when to conceive and how to avoid conception. This work will continue to help women throughout the world understand and better control their bodies.

Janet E. Smith, Ph.D.
Chair of Life Ethics, Prof. of Moral Theology, Sacred Heart Major Seminary, Detroit, Michigan

Mercedes WIlson's teaching materials on Natural Family Planning are unsurpassed for their clarity and blessed simplicity. She has done the world a remarkable service in developing instructional aids that help any couple the world over, from the illiterate to the most learned, to learn the mechanics of NFP. It has been proven time and again that her method works and that those who use it achieve great confidence in the method. The rest of us have an obligation to make these materials known and used as widely as possible.

Joe and Michelle Maher
Michigan

My wife and I were eager to have a child. She became pregnant but miscarried. After the miscarriage, we were afraid that it would be difficult to conceive again since it's been very difficult for the women in my wife's family to conceive. Because of the simplicity and ease of the method we decided to use it to help us. Shortly after we began the method, my wife conceived! We are elated and strongly recommend this method. I am especially enthusiastic about it because of my participation in charting!

Judy Ford
Louisiana

I was introduced to the Ovulation Method after five years of taking the Pill. For 20 years now my husband and I have been using the method to avoid pregnancy and to conceive our two children. If I had known about this method before, the Pill would never have been considered and I would not have suffered side-effects from using it. It's time that women are made aware that there is an alternative which is natural and effective.

Greg and Natia Meehan
Virginia

By using this method, our marriage is more unified because we work together and have come to an understanding of the wondrous nature of both man and woman. Sharing responsibility for our combined fertility has been just as unifying as the marital act itself.

Dr. Marie T. Gould, D.N.Sc., RN
The Johns Hopkins Hospital

Mastery of the Ovulation Method places control of fertility not with the physician, not with the nurse, but where it belongs, with the married couple. Only in this way are the couple respected as autonomous individuals.

Jorge and Eugenia Gonzalez
Mexico, D. F.

The greatest gift any newly married couple could have is the knowledge of human sexuality as presented in your book. Your video and book are our constant source of consultation.

Thomas Mwangi
Muranga, Kenya

Thank Mercedes Wilson, she has freed many couples from contraceptive prison. Muranga being populated with farmers, it is quite easy for the couples to relate fertile phase with the rainy season and infertile phase with the dry season.

Dr. Linan Chang
Prof. of Ob-Gyn
Shanghai, China

If it is compared with other methods, I think the advantages of the Ovulation Method is that it is natural. It is natural for human beings.

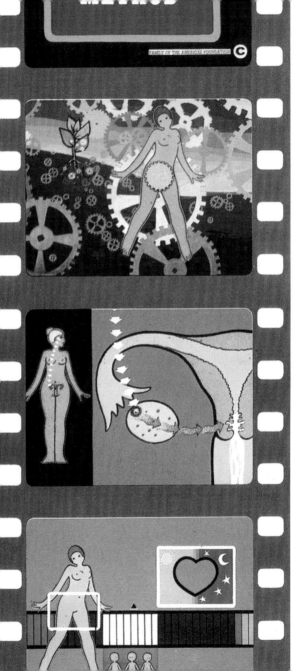

Educational Materials from Family of the Americas

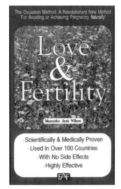

LOVE & FERTILITY VIDEO/DVD - produced by a team of international experts - corresponds to this book. 30 minutes. Available in NTSC, PAL, SECAM, 1/2"; English, Spanish and many other languages.

CHARTING KIT - The most essential part of learning the Ovulation Method is keeping a daily chart of the woman's cycle. This complete permanent record-keeping charting kit comes with a 6 month chart, full-color photo stamps, and observation instructions.

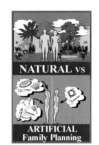

VIDEO/DVD
NATURAL VS. ARTIFICIAL FAMILY PLANNING
Women from around the world discuss their personal experience with artificial birth control, including detailed descriptions of the side effects that they have endured. Also includes an explanation of the Ovulation Method of Natural Family Planning and summarizes the benefits of using natural methods.

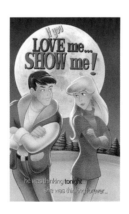

VIDEO/DVD, BOOK or CD-ROM
"If You LOVE me...SHOW me!" is an animated video about two teenagers and how they handle their tested commitment to chastity. Young people will realize that the decisions they make today will affect them for a lifetime. How do they know they're really in love? How do they show it? How far is too far? Fast-paced and entertaining, this is an engaging story about moral convictions and the courage to stand by them. The companion full-color resource book can be used by teens, parents, and teachers. This story is also available in an interactive CD ROM which includes a fun-filled game to test the teen's comprehension of the very important message of chastity.

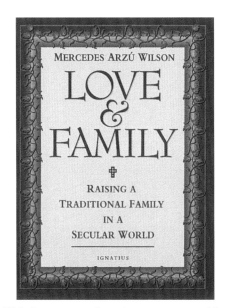

MERCEDES ARZÚ WILSON

LOVE & FAMILY

☩

RAISING A
TRADITIONAL FAMILY
IN A
SECULAR WORLD

IGNATIUS

This is a comprehensive resource guide written by a parent for parents, and educators who work with children, and includes the experience of the most outstanding leaders in scientific, social and religious sectors. Its family centered approach combines extensive references with practical suggestions to empower parents who wish to reclaim their positions as the primary educators of their children, especially in the field of human sexuality. This book displays the tools parents need to guide and protect their children by enriching their knowledge with the latest statistical evidence presented in simple, easy to understand graphs. They will become knowledgeable in the field of anatomy and physiology and they will attain the positive knowledge of the most advanced scientific and practical methods of Natural Family Planning. With the tools and knowledge provided here, parents will better understand their child's needs at every age level, and will confidently be able to assist their children in their physical, moral and spiritual growth and development.

Includes 48 color illustrations.

"Your work with the families is so important. If there is no peace in the world today, it is because there is no peace in the family. Help your families to make their homes centers of compassion and forgive constantly and so bring peace. Your first duty is to be a family."
Blessed Mother Teresa, MC

"Happy are the children whose parents read this book and put into action these counsels. The children will be preserved from venereal disease, including AIDS, they will be told the truth: There is no such thing as safe sex in promiscuity."
Jerome Lejeune, M.D., Ph.D.
Discoverer of the genetic basis
of Down's Syndrome

"A remarkable achievement and a wonderful piece of work—pulling all this together."
Walker Percy, M.D.

"The information and wisdom provided here will help families guide their children toward health and away from the misinformation and confusion toward sexuality that characterizes this last decade of the twentieth century."
Armand M. Nicholi, Jr., M.D.
Professor of Psychiatry,
Harvard Medical School

Acknowledgements

I would like to express my appreciation to the many people who helped me with this book. These include:

- The late William Carrigan of Kensington, Maryland, whose extensive experience provided invaluable advice.

- Drs. John and Evelyn Billings of Melbourne, Australia, who developed the Ovulation Method and it is still being taught throughout the world.

- The late Dr. James Brown, Professor, Department of Obstetrics and Gynecology at the University of Melbourne, Australia, who, through his collaborative research, has provided much of the scientific support for the Ovulation Method and this book.

- Dr. Henry Burger, Director, Medical Research Center, Prince Henry's Hospital, Melbourne, Australia, who, through his collaborative research has also provided much of the scientific support for the Ovulation Method.

- Dr. Erik Odeblad, Professor and Chairman of the Department of Medical Biophysics, the New University of Umea, Sweden, who, through his pioneering research on cervical mucus, has done much to advance medical knowledge on the structure and function of cervical mucus as it relates to fertility and infertility.

- Sr. Anna Cappela, M.D., Drs. Elena Giacchi and Valeria Navarretta of Rome, Italy, who provided much of the scientific guidance of the text for the film from which this book was originally developed.

- The late Dr. Ruth Taylor, who worked as Medical Director, Natural Family Planning, St. Francis Hospital, Wichita, Kansas, who contributed scientific information to this book and whose advice and editing guided me through its development.

- Dr. John Brennan and his wonderful wife, Joan, of Milwaukee, Wisconsin, who so faithfully contributed to this work.

- Paul A. Byrne, M.D. and Walt Weaver, M.D. whose friendship and advice I appreciate so much.

- Angela Lanfranchi, M.D., brilliant scientist who is a dedicated contributor to the health of women and has shared invaluable knowledge to this book.

- Fr. William Ryan, S.J., who has provided valuable contributions to our book and to the Hispanic community of Maryland, Virginia and Washington, D.C.

- Sr. Francesca Kearns, Ph.D., Fr. Denis St. Marie and the late Fr. William Gibbons, M.D., whose missionary teaching in Central and South America provided many of the ideas in the development of this book.

- Luigi Turolla of Rome, Italy, whose brilliant ideas and illustrations have enhanced this book, and for his patience and untiring dedication to the Foundation's work.

- Fr. Daniel McCaffrey, for his life-long dedication to the promotion of Natural Family Planning throughout the United States and Europe.

- Marjorie Harrigan of Houston, Texas, former Director of the Natural Family Planning Clinic, South Texas Family Planning and Health Corporation, who helped me develop the text of this book and whose advice I greatly valued throughout the years.

- Tom and Rosi Cunningham, whose constant support and expertise have been invaluable to the development of the Ovulation Method Charting Coach and Nature's Method CD-ROM.

- The late Dr. Herbert Ratner of Oak Park, Illinois, for his great wisdom and advice over the years.

- Alberto and Christine Vollmer of Caracas, Venezuela, for their continued support over the years.

- The late Msgr. Charles Fortier, for his steadfast commitment to the Hispanic community of California in promoting the Ovulation Method.

- The late Anne Higgins of Washington, D.C., whose encouragement and experience together with her late husband George were invaluable to our work.

- Dr. John Bruchalski, OB-GYN, for his dedication to the health of women and the welfare of the family by promoting the Ovulation Method in his Clinic and throughout various states in the United States.

- *The late Ringold Olivier of Mandeville, Louisiana, who showed constant dedication, loyalty and friendship since I first began this work.*

- *The late Walker Percy, to whom I owe more gratitude than words can express for his support, advice and encouragement in writing this book.*

- *Family of the Americas teaching staff dedicated to giving their time and talents wherever we're needed to train the clergy, sisters, lay people, including medical professionals. These stars include Judith Leonard, Luis and Marta Oseguera, Dr. Pilar Calva, Nancy Budowski, K.C. Schnitker, Doug Scott.*

- *The many volunteers who have so generously helped us over the years. Including Delaine Johnson, Kay Cole, Faith Torsani whose support and dedication is invaluable to the success of our work.*

- *Douglas Scott whose support has been unending in the editing of this book.*

- *To our faithful teachers around the world, especially Josefina Camou, Janet Bettcher, Mary Beth Biese, Karla Boy, Dominique de Quiñones, Paula Damasio, Dora Marina Monterroso de Chew, Ana Maria de Socoreque, Dolores Sotz, Maria Sotz and the many thousands that would be impossible to mention in this book.*

- *My staff of Brenda Williams, Mary Resinck and Nancy Budowski, our new Executive Director whose work and enthusiasm becomes contagious around the office. Her editing advice has been invaluable in this new addition. Louisa Woolery , whose wisdom in design and layout of this new addition has been invaluable. I could never thank them enough for their untiring dedication and cheerful willingness to work long hours including weekends and holidays. Without their commitment, this work would not be available worldwide.*

- *With deep gratitude to Family of the Americas Board of Directors, especially Robert and Joan Smith, Patricia Lynch, Gerald and Bette Hoag, Judith Leonard, Joni and Steve Abdalla, for their faithful and constant support of our work.*

- *Finally, my family, whose patience, understanding, and support have made my work possible.*